RESTRUCTURING THE MEDICAL PROFESSION

STATE OF HEALTH SERIES

Edited by Chris Ham, Professor of Health Policy and Management at the University of Birmingham and Director of the Strategy Unit at the Department of Health.

Current and forthcoming titles

RESTRUCTURING THE MEDICAL PROFESSION:
The Intraprofessional Relations of GPs and Hospital Consultants

Juan I Baeza

Open University Press

Open University Press
McGraw-Hill Education
McGraw-Hill House
Shoppenhangers Road
Maidenhead
Berkshire
SL6 2QL
United Kingdom

Email: enquiries@openup.co.uk
World wide web: www.openup.co.uk

and
Two Penn Plaza, New York, NY 10121-2289, USA

First published 2005

A catalogue record of this book is available from the British Library

ISBN–10: 0 335 21627 7 (pb)   0 335 21628 5 (hb)
ISBN–13: 9780 335 216227 (pb)   9780 335 216284 (hb)

Library of Congress Cataloging-in-Publication Data
CIP data has been applied for

Typeset by RefineCatch Limited, Bungay, Suffolk
Printed in Great Britain by Bell & Bain Ltd, Glasgow

To Debbie, Alfie and Freya

CONTENTS

SERIES EDITOR'S INTRODUCTION

Health services in many developed countries have come under critical scrutiny in recent years. In part this is because of increasing expenditure, much of it funded from public sources, and the pressure this has put on governments seeking to control public spending. Also important has been the perception that resources allocated to health services are not always deployed in an optimal fashion. Thus at a time when the scope for increasing expenditure is extremely limited, there is a need to search for ways of using existing budgets more efficiently. A further concern has been the desire to ensure access to health care of various groups on an equitable basis. In some countries this has been linked to a wish to enhance patient choice and to make service providers more responsive to patients as consumers.

Underlying these specific concerns are a number of more fundamental developments which have a significant bearing on the performance of health services. Three are worth highlighting. First, there are demographic changes, including the ageing population and the decline in the proportion of the population of working age. These changes will both increase the demand for health care and at the same time limit the ability of health services to respond to this demand.

Second, advances in medical science will also give rise to new demands within the health services. These advances cover a range of possibilities, including innovations in surgery, drug therapy, screening and diagnosis. The pace of innovation quickened as the end of the twentieth century approached, with significant implications for the funding and provision of services.

Third, public expectations of health services are rising as those who use services demand higher standards of care. In part, this is stimulated by developments within the health service, including the availability of new technology. More fundamentally, it stems from the emergence of a more educated and informed population, in which people are accustomed to being treated as consumers rather than patients.

Against this background, policy makers in a number of countries are reviewing the future of health services. Those countries which have traditionally relied on a market in health care are making greater use of regulation and planning. Equally, those countries which have traditionally relied on regulation and planning are moving towards a more competitive approach. In no country is there complete satisfaction with existing methods of financing and delivery, and everywhere there is a search for new policy instruments.

The aim of this series is to contribute to debate about the future of health services through an analysis of major issues in health policy. These issues have been chosen because they are both of current interest and of enduring importance. The series is intended to be accessible to students and informed lay readers as well as to specialists working in this field. The aim is to go beyond a textbook approach to health policy analysis and to encourage authors to move debate about their issues forward. In this sense, each book presents a summary of current research and thinking, and an exploration of future policy directions.

Professor Chris Ham
Professor of Health Policy and Management at the University of Birmingham

ACKNOWLEDGEMENTS

The material in this book is based on several years' work. While I was at the University of Kent my colleagues Mike Calnan and John Butler gave me valuable advice and the encouragement I needed. I would also like to express my gratitude to Steve Harrison and Andy Alaszewski for their extensive comments and suggestions on earlier work that has formed the basis of this book. I am also grateful to all those who agreed to be interviewed during the course of this research.

This publication is supported by a grant from the Research and Graduate Studies Committee, Faculty of Arts, The University of Melbourne.

1

RESTRUCTURING PROFESSIONAL RELATIONS: HEALTH REFORM AND THE MEDICAL PROFESSION

INTRODUCTION

This chapter will provide the policy context for the book as a whole. The historical development of the British medical profession is examined, the evolution of the two branches of medicine is analysed both before and after the creation of the National Health Service (NHS). The influence that general practitioners (GPs) and hospital consultants have had on health policy, how policies have impacted upon them and how these developments have influenced their intra-professional relations is then examined. The differing development of GPs and hospital consultants within the NHS is analysed, providing an account of the evolution of intraprofessional relations of GPs and hospital consultants within the NHS.

THE POLICY BACKGROUND

There have been numerous studies of managers and management within the NHS, which have examined their impact upon the health service (see Harrison, Hunter, Marnoch and Pollitt, 1992 for a review of such studies). Some of these empirical studies have explored the relationships between doctors and managers, examining how the introduction of management into the NHS affected the balance of power between managers and doctors. However, the intraprofes-sional relations within the medical profession in the British NHS have been relatively neglected by empirical research. Often the medical profession has been viewed as a relatively homogenous whole, ignoring the various tensions that exist within this varied professional group. There have been historical studies of the two main branches of medicine – hospital doctors and GPs – within the British health care system that have illustrated their differing fortunes before and after the formation of the NHS. Honigsbaum (1979) pointed out how health policies often impacted on the two branches in quite different ways, as the example of the formation of the NHS in the United Kingdom illustrates. This has continued to be true for health policies that have been introduced more recently.

GPs and primary care in general have undergone many important changes in the past decade. These have included two new contracts for GPs since 1990 (Department of Health, 1989a; Department of Health, 2003b) and general practitioner fundholding (Department of Health, 1989b). Added to these has been the clear emphasis placed upon primary care in various government documents such as *The Health of the Nation* and *Shifting the Balance of Power* (Department of Health, 1992; Department of Health, 2001c), policies aimed at primary care-led commissioning, and more recently the creation of primary care groups (PCGs) and then primary care trusts (PCTs) (Department of Health, 1997). The hospital sector has also undergone large and rapid changes at the same time; many of these have had an impact on the hospital consultants working in this area. These changes have included the introduction of general management in the 1980s (Griffiths, 1983), the transfer of consultant contracts from regional to individual hospital trust level (Department of Health, 1989c), the implementation of medical audit (Department of Health, 1989d), resource management (Department of Health, 1989e), the general impact of contracting with the creation of the NHS internal market (Department of Health, 1989f), the introduction of clinical governance to both secondary and primary care (Department of Health, 1998) and more recently the implementation of a new consultant contract (Department of Health, 2004c).

The internal market, in theory at least, meant that provider units would have to win contracts in order to remain viable; and as a consequence hospital consultants needed contracts from purchasers to preserve their jobs. Within this market environment GPs became either direct purchasers (as part of a fundholding practice) or more closely involved in purchasing with health authorities (as part of locality commissioning teams). It was they who were in a position to exert pressures on providers and thus upon the hospital consultants who work within them. It is easy to think that such pressures were wholly novel to the NHS, so it is worth noting that these changes have had a history within the NHS. Over two decades ago, long before the creation of the internal market, similar competitive potentials were perceived to be present. Jeffreys and Sachs (1983) reported on a study where a hospital consultant explained why he was keen to hold clinics at health centres as well as at the hospital:

> *It's not elegant or attractive, but a fact of life in London that if one hospital doesn't get the [health] Centre patients the others will, and I don't want my department closed down. So it's important I satisfy the practices with the services I provide.* (p. 63)

However, these competitive pressures were heightened with the introduction of the internal market into the NHS in 1991. The attempted replacement of the previous hierarchical and bureaucratic structures by market mechanisms could potentially alter the balance of power within the medical profession.

The politically driven changes that have occurred within the NHS have sought to achieve greater value for money by introducing business-like thinking and an enhancement of the managerial capacity within the health system in order to reduce the power of the professions (Ferlie, 1997). These health care reforms have had an impact on the roles and relationships within the NHS, which in turn have influenced the health care system as a whole. Ferlie (1997) argues that this theme of changing roles, relationships and power balances that has been investigated by researchers can be traced back to Alford's *Health Care Politics* published in 1975. Researchers who have examined this theme have devoted their attention to the impact that the introduction of general management has had on the roles and relationships within the NHS and to what extent it has challenged the dominance of the medical profession (Harrison, 1994; Harrison, Hunter, Marnoch and Pollitt, 1992; Pettigrew, Ferlie and McKee, 1992; Strong and Robinson, 1990). However, the dominant position of doctors within the NHS makes the medical profession arguably the most important player within this complex organization. Researchers have relatively neglected the impact that the various rounds of health reforms have had *within* the medical profession.

THE RISE OF THE BRITISH MEDICAL PROFESSION

As Britain entered the twentieth century, its health care system was largely private with some charitable and public provision for the so-called 'deserving poor'. Hospital doctors would be willing to treat poor patients on a charitable basis in voluntary hospitals if they presented with 'interesting', acute and treatable conditions. It was not until the end of the nineteenth century that the hospital began to grow as the central location for medical treatment. The introduction of antiseptic surgery in 1865 followed by anaesthetics in 1875 allowed the hospital to take centre stage within the health care system. During the nineteenth century, physicians treated their clients either in their own homes or in the doctor's surgery. Throughout most of the nineteenth century, hospitals were likely to do more harm than good and therefore they were utilized only by the urban poor who had no other alternative. During the twentieth century, as medicine became more complex, then so the hospital grew in importance. The voluntary hospitals became the power bases for the elite physicians and surgeons (Hollingsworth, 1986).

It was the 1858 Medical Act that allowed the medical profession to ring-fence itself against unqualified practitioners by creating the General Medical Council (GMC) as the profession's registering body. This Act proved to be very successful in limiting the number of registered doctors: the 1841 census contained 30,000 doctors while the first medical directories that began in 1853 contained only 11,000 entries (Allsop, 1995). Following the unification of the medical profession, it was the consultants and their royal colleges who largely dictated the direction of the profession as a whole. As the hospital grew in importance the better-organized hospital consultants could shape medical education in their favour and centre it on hospital practice (Parry and Parry, 1976).

The hospital consultants were highly autonomous since, as most of the cases they treated in the hospital were charitable, their patients made few demands on them. The hospital consultants' income was mainly derived from their fee-paying patients who were treated either in the patient's home or in the doctor's office. The hospital was important to consultants because it was from the hospital networks, such as the hospitals' board of trustees, that they derived their wealthy fee-paying clients. General practitioners were successfully kept out of these networks and as a consequence their clientele came from the less wealthy middle and lower classes (Hollingsworth, 1986).

The GPs' working life was quite different to that of the hospital consultant. The GP had no access to the voluntary hospitals and derived a much lower income by treating poorer patients. GPs had to compete among themselves and the more prestigious physicians in order to treat patients. Due to the similarity in the roles of physician and GP there was a considerable amount of poaching of patients between these two groups. GPs were thus reluctant to refer their patients on to consultants for fear of their patient being poached and thus depriving the GP of income. The British Medical Association (BMA) recognized this problem and sought to order the market relationship of doctors by putting in place the referral system between GPs and consultants. The BMA called on the GMC to police the intraprofessional rivalry by applying its rules, which did not allow advertising of services or the disparagement of fellow doctors (Hollingsworth, 1986). The divide between the GP and the hospital doctor was made clear and explicit.

The GPs were far less autonomous than their hospital colleagues. Many of the GPs' patients were members of friendly societies, which were important organizations within health care prior to the creation of the NHS. The members of the friendly societies paid a small regular sum of money for which they could receive treatment from a GP. The friendly societies were effectively the employers of the GPs and had the power to determine their work. By the end of the nineteenth and early twentieth century the GPs' professional dominance and autonomy was low. The GPs resented effectively being employed by the friendly societies and wanted to be freed from their control. Prompted by the worsening relationship between the friendly societies and GPs the BMA began to campaign against a system which GPs saw as detrimental to them both economically and professionally. This campaign was one of the factors that contributed to the creation of the 1911 National Health Insurance (NHI) Act (Hollingsworth, 1986).

The state's involvement in primary care greatly improved the GPs' position and weakened that of friendly societies, while the GPs proved to be well organized during their negotiations with the state in setting up the new NHI system. The *British Medical Journal* at the time summed up the doctors' strength rather neatly, arguing that: '*The country could perhaps do without Mr Lloyd George, but it could not do without the doctors. That is the strength of our position*' (quoted in Parry and Parry, 1976, p. 190). The NHI Act meant that the GPs had greater control over their work and were not so heavily reliant on the friendly societies.

Although status differences between the two branches of medicine remained, the new NHI system succeeded in raising the income and the status of the GP. Moreover, it meant that the hospital consultants were now dependent on the GPs for referrals, forcing the consultants to cultivate good relationships with the GPs. However, the Royal College of Physicians prohibited their members from entering into partnerships with GPs, thus preventing closer ties developing between the two branches of medicine.

As the hospital became the centre for medical care then so the status and influence of the hospital doctor increased. GPs saw the expanding hospital sector as a potential threat and they unsuccessfully tried to restrict patients' access to the hospitals' outpatient services. For their part the hospitals successfully expanded their outpatient services to increase their finances by treating more hospital insurance policy holders. This situation created a sharp tension between the two branches of medicine as more fee-paying middle-class patients began to utilize the growing hospital services instead of the services of GPs. The clear separation between the GP and the hospital consultant that NHI had helped exacerbate created a disunited and weakened profession, a disunity that was to be exploited in order to create the NHS.

The development of medical care throughout the twentieth century was influenced predominately by the elite hospital consultants. One of the ways that they achieved this domination was through their control of medical education and research. Both medical education and research have largely been centred on the hospital, while general practice has until quite recently been sidelined. Ill health was defined (and to a certain extent is still defined) as being micro-causal and purely biological in nature, and it was this view that shaped the provision of health care. As medical education and research form the basis of the development of medicine, the fact that hospital doctors have managed to dominate this field is an important factor in the development of the two branches of medicine in terms of their influence. Maintaining hospital medicine at the centre of medical research and education has ensured hospital doctors' dominance within the medical profession hierarchy, while structural changes involved in creating the National Health Service were to further enhance their position.

THE CREATION OF THE NHS

The Second World War brought the inadequacies of the British health care system into sharp relief. The large civilian casualties anticipated by the war prompted the government to establish the Emergency Medical Service (EMS) in 1939 as part of the Ministry of Health. The EMS took over the running of many of the existing hospitals and the hospital consultants became active in setting it up and running the service. Many consultants reduced or gave up their private practice in order to participate in the EMS as salaried employees. The experience of the EMS helped alert the hospital doctors to the need for government planning in the area of health care.

The structure of the NHS, which was created in 1948, was heavily based on the wishes of Britain's economic and social elite. On the one hand, the medical profession saw that the pre-NHS structures were unsustainable and foresaw that an NHS fashioned by them offered them great opportunities for advancement. On the other hand, the state felt that it needed to provide its citizens with a health service that was more egalitarian and efficient than what was available at that time and to do this it needed the support of the medical profession; a concordat between the medical profession and the state had to be struck. The highly centralized structure of the NHS allowed the hospital consultant elite and their royal colleges easily to penetrate the centres of power and to influence the agendas and discussions regarding health policy.

When the concept of a National Health Service was raised in 1942 there was a general agreement from all sectors of the profession; the disagreements emerged as the negotiations on the details of such a service developed. A BMA poll on the 1944 White Paper gave an indication of the feelings of the medical profession towards the establishment of an NHS: there was a small majority (53 per cent) who were against the creation of the NHS as outlined in the White Paper, but 60 per cent were in favour of the creation of a completely free and comprehensive health service (Forsyth, 1973). These results illustrate the fact that there was a general agreement on the establishment of a 'free at the point of use' health service, although there was less agreement on what shape this service should take. The interested parties consisted of the government, the medical profession, the voluntary hospitals and the local authorities. However, in practice the key relationship was the one between the state and the medical profession, more accurately between the state and the two sections of the medical profession: the hospital consultants and the general practitioners (Allsop, 1995).

The then Minister of Health, Aneurin Bevan, felt that the hospital sector was the key to the creation of an NHS. Initially it was envisaged that the local authorities would run the hospitals, as they were already experienced in this prior to the creation of the NHS. However, many doctors resisted this option as they associated local authorities with the under-funded hospital system that had existed up to then, which provided them with few opportunities for their professional advancement. GPs also feared coming under the control of the local authorities – they felt that their professional autonomy would be further threatened if they were to become salaried employees. Consultants who had experienced life as salaried employees in the EMS were less concerned by this prospect and could see the advantages of such a system. Their main concern was to retain their right to maintain a private practice alongside any NHS work. Thus the negotiations surrounding the setting up of the NHS saw the medical profession divided between the hospital doctors on one hand and the GPs on the other: they had different concerns and were unable collectively to put forward a coherent plan of their own.

Bevan exploited this division within the medical profession to enable him to create the NHS. He decided to enlist the support of the most powerful section of the medical profession as he saw it. He therefore sought to gain the support of the royal colleges who were the main representatives of the hospital consultants, as the BMA was seen as representing the GPs. This strategy allowed the hospital consultants to gain many concessions from Bevan in exchange for their support in the setting up of the NHS. The consultants managed to secure the retention of their private practice, a high degree of control over appointments and promotions and control of the merit award system. Thus, giving the royal colleges a powerful voice on the development of the service was the reward for their co-operation in the creation of the NHS. The GPs for their part also achieved important concessions – they managed to retain their independent contractor status and their income did improve as a result of the NHS. The NHS structure allowed the medical profession, largely in the shape of hospital consultants, to decide on local resource allocations while the state set the global health budget. The new NHS was to be professionally dominated; Parry and Parry (1976) stated that:

> *The nationalisation of the hospitals and the re-organisation of general practice eventuated in a profession-dominated National Health Service which achieved for the medical profession a constitutional position in the realm matched only by the Church and the Law.* (p. 208)

When one considers the balance sheet, it is clear that the biggest winners within the medical profession were the hospital consultants. They had the prospect of working in well-equipped and well-resourced hospitals that excluded the GPs and they could retain their lucrative private practices. The consultants' junior staff allowed them to be part-time employees of the NHS and gave them the freedom to engage in their private practice. This was an option that was taken by two-thirds of consultants in 1959 (Hollingsworth, 1986), as pursuing a private practice gave consultants increased status and income.

THE DEVELOPMENT OF THE MEDICAL PROFESSION WITHIN THE NHS

Following the establishment of the NHS GPs witnessed deterioration in their status within the medical profession, both economically in terms of salary and politically in terms of their influence on the service (Forsyth, 1973). A few years after the creation of the NHS a gap in terms of status and income had again appeared between hospital doctors and GPs. The GP was a generalist at a time when the specialist was highly valued; the GP had little contact with the hospital which was the focus of medical advancement; expansions were being planned for the hospital sector and not in general practice; and the hospital doctors had their royal colleges while the GPs did not. The hospital doctors' income was considerably higher than that of the GP and could be increased even further by engaging in private practice. By 1956 the median annual income of the hospital consultant was £3,130 while that of the GP was just £2,160 (Parry and Parry, 1976).

Although GPs earned more than hospital doctors upon entry, once hospital doctors became consultants their earning potential over a lifetime was much greater than that of GPs (Forsyth, 1973). Another one of the GPs' concerns was that they were offered no financial assistance to improve their surgeries or employ ancillary staff. Large GP patient workloads also meant that they found it difficult to spare any time for their professional development. The new College of General Practitioners and the BMA lobbied government to improve the situation of GPs. The government responded to these calls by reaching a settlement in 1966 with the BMA on its call for a Family Doctor's Charter (BMA, 1965) which called for financial improvements that were aimed at making becoming a GP more attractive. Another boost to general practice was given by the 1968 Royal Commission on Medical Education, which agreed with the Royal College of General Practitioners' calls for a qualifying exam for all new entrants into general practice. It was felt that such reforms would raise the quality of general practice and thereby raise the status of the GP. This same Royal Commission also made the recommendation, which was accepted, to make general practice a compulsory part of a medical student's training.

The separation between GPs and hospital doctors that had existed before the NHS and was compounded by the creation of the NHS would continue to create problems in the future. Sir John Maude, a member of the committee that produced the Guillebaud Report, articulated the problems:

> *The mischief to which the division of the service gives rise falls broadly under two heads, (a) the administrative divorce of curative from preventative medicine and of general practice from hospital practice and the overlaps, gaps and confusion caused thereby and (b) the predominant position of the hospital service and the consequent danger of general practice and preventative and social medicine falling into the background.* (Quoted in Allsop, 1995, p. 44)

Thus, only a few years after the creation of NHS there was a great divide between the two branches of medicine, which had a structural and historical basis. However, it was not only the hospital consultants who were successful in professional advancement within the new NHS structure; in the years following the creation of the NHS the GPs managed to regain some of the ground that had been lost to their hospital consultant colleagues.

THE RENAISSANCE OF GENERAL PRACTICE

A decade after the creation of the NHS there was no designated postgraduate training for those entering general practice. To become a hospital consultant on the other hand one had to pass difficult specialist exams that many failed. Doctors entering general practice were taught almost exclusively using the hospital model. Gray (1979) has argued that

> *the message from the medical schools, both implicitly and explicitly, was that the best medicine was practised in hospitals and the best of all in teaching hospitals . . . General practice in Britain is still the dustbin of medicine.* (pp. 2–3)

This situation began to change only slowly. First, in 1950 the BMA stated in the Cohen Committee Report that there was a need for three years' specific vocational training for those wishing to enter general practice. Second and most importantly, by the creation of the College of General Practitioners in 1952, this had to be established in secret due to specialist opposition (Hunt, 1972). The college received the royal seal of approval and joined the other medical royal colleges in 1967 when it received its royal charter.

GPs needed to be represented in positions where policies were discussed and decided upon. These were positions that the specialists' royal colleges had had access to for many years. It was felt that the absence of GPs in such settings was one of the reasons why this branch of medicine had been sidelined within the NHS. Since the establishment of the college, members have gained representation on important government and medical committees, and commissions thus being able to represent the GP view (Gray, 1992).

An early aim for the college was for GPs to establish posts within the British universities. The intentions were to present general practice to medical students as a different but credible branch of medicine and establish a research base for general practice, something that had been lacking until then. It took 11 years for the first chair in general practice to be established in a British university. The principle objective of the college was to position general practice as a separate and legitimate discipline within medicine. To do this it had to establish an academic autonomy for itself so that general practice could be taught from its own research base as opposed to that of other medical disciplines.

The absence of a research base for general practice was seen as a severe disadvantage to this branch of the profession – a fundamental obstacle to the advancement of general practice. Gray (1992) described GPs in 1952 as

> the oldest branch of medical profession. Yet they did little research, published few papers, rarely taught medical students, had limited opportunities for apprentice-type training, no university department of general practice and no professor of general practice anywhere in the world. (p. 33)

However, the decade between 1960 and 1970 represented a period of professional development for general practice (Cartwright and Anderson, 1979). Their status and income witnessed resurgence – they gained higher average income rises than hospital consultants during this period. A GP's average net income during this decade rose by 103 per cent while that of consultants rose by between 62 and 77 per cent. These rises meant that by 1970 the minimum a consultant would be earning was £4,512, which was less than the average-earning GP on £4,920, although the maximum a consultant could be earning due to the system of merit award was £6,330 (Forsyth, 1973). The improved methods of remuneration that enabled GPs to employ ancillary staff and their considerable rises in personal earnings meant that by the end of the 1970s GPs had managed to greatly improve their position within the medical profession.

As far as government policies toward the medical profession were concerned, to this point they had consisted largely of attempting to persuade the profession to change. By 1980 these tactics were seen to have failed to exert the state's desired influence on the profession and the incoming Conservative government sought new policies. It was to pursue policies of cost containment and value for money in the public services, including the NHS, and there was an increasing desire on the part of consumers for professionals to become more accountable.

2

REFORMING PROFESSIONAL RELATIONS

INTRODUCTION

This chapter will consider the period between 1979 and 2005 in terms of health care policy, which can be divided into three principle stages. The 1980s can be seen as a period of managerialism and the introduction of management techniques that had their origin in the private sector: what has become known as the 'new public management' (NPM) model. The late 1980s and mid 1990s can be represented by the introduction of internal markets and competition into the NHS. With the success of New Labour in the 1997 general election, the late 1990s can be seen as a period where the ideas of co-operation and partnership were reintroduced into the NHS, while still maintaining (and in some cases strengthening) many of the previous administration's market-inspired reforms. This division in health policy is not to say that there were no other policy strands, such as consumerism, during this period or that managerialism ended in 1990, as it is still very much part of the NHS in the new millennium. However, these three historical periods can be discerned from the analysis of health policy during the past two decades.

NEW PUBLIC MANAGEMENT

The make-up of post-World War 2 society was quite different from that of the 1970s and 1980s. For example, in 1951 the proportion of the workforce who were manual workers was nearly two-thirds and by 1981 it was less than half; only just over a quarter of the population owned their own home in 1947 and by 1981 well over half had become home owners and the number was to increase further under the Thatcher administration (Klein, 1995). The more affluent and better-educated public of the 1980s would interact with the state and the medical profession in quite a different way to the deferential and patient public of the 1940s and 1950s. The political environment of the post-war state had substantially altered by the 1980s and 1990s and faced quite different demands in the social policy arena. The creation and subsequent development of an NHS in Britain repre-sented an activist model of the state where state intervention was seen as necessary to avoid the perceived deficiencies and failures of the private market (Minogue, 2000).

However, as Britain entered the fiscal crisis of the early 1970s this activist model of the state came into question. Although it is import-ant to note that the largest cuts in public spending occurred during the Labour administration of 1977–8, the ideological attacks on what was considered an over-activist state were spearheaded by the New Right ideology that was associated with the prime minister, Margaret Thatcher (Clarke, Gewirtz and McLaughlin, 2000). The activist state model was attacked for being inefficient, over-bureaucratic, unresponsive, over-invasive and allowing elite and priv-ileged groups to exploit the system for their own aims (Minogue, 2000). The critics of the activist state argued that the market could provide the solutions to these problems; by introducing market prin-ciples into the welfare state the deficiencies in the system would be addressed. The Conservative government that gained power in 1979 was sympathetic to this emerging free-market thinking and it was also keen to confront what it regarded as the self-serving professions. By the mid-1980s it had already shown its disdain for the teaching and academic professions and it was now ready to do battle with the more powerful professions of law and medicine. By the end of the 1980s one can see a strong state and an empowered consumer generation.

The NPM reforms that began in the late 1970s and that were applied to the NHS in the 1980s advocated various strategies such as reductions in public services and their restructuring via partial or wholesale privatizations, slimming down central services, improving efficiency by contracting out non-core services, and the introduction of internal markets. These new strategies needed to be managed in a different way: public services could not merely be passively adminis-tered, they had to be actively managed so as to bring about these fundamental changes. Public administration had to be transformed into public management. This new form of welfare delivery was described by Butcher (1995) as:

> *A system dominated by central government departments, local authorities and the NHS, and based upon the values and practices of public administration . . . is being replaced by a new set of practices and values, based upon a new language of welfare delivery which emphasizes efficiency and value for money, competition and markets, consumerism and customer care.* (p. 161)

This new form of managerialism consisted of creating professional managers who were given a considerable amount of discretion in order to reach clear goals and objectives; and their rewards, both personal and organizational, would be closely linked to specific levels of performance (Hood, 1991). The NPM took on many guises within the NHS, ranging from marginal initiatives such as contracting out hospitals' non-core services such as laundry and cleaning to more fundamental ones such as the introduction of general management.

MANAGEMENT ENTERS THE NHS

The first practical articulations of this new philosophy within the NHS appeared in 1983 with the introduction of compulsory competitive tendering (CCT) and general management. These first two manifestations of the NPM model were to signify not just a change in the content of policy but also a change in the delivery and style of policy. As with many of the new policies directed at the public services, their impact was far from dramatic: the National Audit Office (1987) calculated that by 1986 the CCT policy had yielded only £86 million in annual savings. However, the directive mode of implementation by the centre showed that the new government was not prepared to be deflected from implementing a new *modus operandi* for the NHS.

The introduction of general management into the NHS was seen at the time as a major development. It followed a 25-page report compiled by four people in six months (Klein, 1995). The accidental chairman of the inquiry, Sir Roy Griffiths (as he was later to become), was at the time managing director of the successful supermarket chain Sainsbury's. Long and highly consultative royal commissions were no longer necessary: what the NHS needed was a management consultant from the private sector to advise the service on how to reform. The diagnosis was not new but it was short and to the point: the service was suffering from *institutional stagnation*. The report recommended that most of the service's ills could be cured by a strong dose of management. As a result of the report's recommendations a new management structure was introduced into the NHS, with managers placed at every level of the service.

The new managers were given clear incentives to drive through change as their salaries and jobs depended on them making the necessary changes to improve performance. However, as with so many national policies, implementation at a local level seldom resembled the authors' wishes. The change from passive and consensually based administration to assertive and directive management was to be a slow and, many would say, unsuccessful process in the NHS (Harrison, Hunter, Marnoch and Pollitt, 1992). However, many of the new managers relished the opportunity to use their new powers (or at least what they saw as their new powers) to challenge professional interests within the NHS, particularly those of the hospital consultants.

It was not only the recommendations themselves that the profession objected to but also their style and origin. It was not so much the substance of the report that was momentous, as many of the points it raised were not new and the previous royal commission on the NHS which reported in 1979 had recognized the problems of leadership that the Griffiths report re-identified. It was, rather, the language used in the recommendations that was quite different; it spoke of *products, customers* and *levels of quality*. The introduction of general management into the NHS can thus be seen as an attempt to bring about a cultural change rather than a structural one (Mark and Scott, 1992). Previously these factors had been unquestioned, as professionals could be trusted implicitly to provide the appropriate level and type of care to their patients, and their activities did not need to be actively managed to achieve this. Furthermore, not only did they not need to be managed in this pursuit, they *could not* be managed, as the only people who could discuss the types and standards of medical care were fellow doctors. Administrators, as many doctors still called the new NHS managers, had no legitimate place in such discussions. Before the Griffiths report, relationships within the NHS were based on trust, and this was as true between doctors and patients as it was between doctors and administrators (Hunter, 1998). These mutual relationships were based on implicit obligations that were not precisely defined and decisions were taken consensually rather than in a directive manner. However, the new low-trust relationships needed to become more explicit and codified. Greater definition led to new notions of quality assurance, which entered the NHS lexicon in the mid-1980s as an issue that would become a policy goal, taking centre stage in subsequent reforms. However, by the end of the 1980s it was clear that the rules that governed the supermarket industry – where staff could easily be managed and where their customers were sovereign and free to choose among a host of different providers – could not easily be imported into a health care system that was staffed by powerful professional groups and accessed by information-poor consumers. Although the real impacts of the Griffiths report upon the NHS were minimal, its philosophical attack on the, up to then, unquestioned principles of the NHS was to have a greater impact and would set the necessary foundations for future more radical reforms of the service.

The introduction of management in the 1980s was to be the beginning of a new management culture that would later engulf the medical profession. Although less than a fifth of the new management positions were taken up by doctors in the post-Griffiths NHS (Harrison and Pollitt, 1994), many doctors have now become quasi-managers within the health service in the shape of medical or clinical directors in the hospital sector and GP fundholding leads and PCT board members within primary care. The two developments of compulsory competitive tendering and the introduction of general management described above indirectly impacted upon hospital doctors but the new market-friendly government was not yet ready to tackle the medical profession head on. It had so far concentrated its actions upon the environment within which doctors operated. However, by the end of the 1980s it would tackle the profession head on, as it was time to turn its attentions to primary care.

MANAGING PRIMARY CARE

For a government determined to tackle public expenditure, the open-ended budget of general practice was an obvious target. With a decrease in GP list sizes and an increase in GPs' use of ancillary staff, expenditure on the family practitioner services had escalated faster than any other part of the NHS, with their slice of the financial cake growing from 22 per cent in 1979–80 to 24 per cent in 1985–86 (Klein, 1995). The government's first port of call within primary care was to be prescribing. The DHSS tackled the rising costs of general practice prescribing by issuing a 'limited list' at the end of 1984. Although the government compromised on some of the details of this policy, its substance remained and thus managed successfully to impinge upon one section of the medical profession's fiercely guarded clinical autonomy.

Further reform was to be undertaken in the area of primary care towards the end of the 1980s. The government's aims for primary care reform were to increase managerial control of these services and to empower patients (Department of Health, 1986). The discussion document also contained policies aimed at strengthening the arm of Family Practitioner Committees (FPCs) which until then had been little more than pay roll offices for GPs. As with the Griffiths reforms in secondary care, weak administration was to be replaced by dynamic management. These new terms and conditions for GPs were imposed upon the profession in 1990 (Department of Health, 1989a) despite the fact that more than 70 per cent of GPs rejected the new contract (Allsop, 1995). The imposition of a new contract upon GPs represented what was to be the first in a new phase of policy making within the NHS that was to see the state asserting a new level of dominance upon the service (Light, 2001). This exercise in primary care showed that the government was willing to confront the medical profession, particularly one section of it, and to impose policy changes upon it that it felt were necessary. The medical profession's previous tactics of blocking, or at least drastically modifying, government policies were proving to be less effective against a government that was prepared to implement health policy in spite of medical opposition.

Although the various Conservative governments had been successful in introducing a greater level of management into the NHS, both at the hospital and primary care level, the impact upon the medical profession itself was less far-reaching. NHS managers were finding it difficult to exert their authority over a profession that was all too ready to hide behind its cloak of expert knowledge. The political nature of an organization such as the NHS was also making life difficult for NHS managers. Politicians were eager to give managers the freedom and power to implement change within the service but were also keen to interfere when changes occurred that were seen as politically unhelpful. Thus, it could be seen that many of the private-sector inspired policies for the NHS were not having the desired effects upon such a professionally dominant and politically sensitive organization. It is perhaps for these reasons among others that a decade of Conservative administration was to end in a crescendo for the NHS in the form of the 1989 White Paper *Working for Patients* (Department of Health, 1989g).

Before going on to consider the impact of the 1991 NHS reforms it is necessary to examine the state of the two branches of medicine and their intraprofessional relations at the dawn of these reforms. The history of the two branches of the medical profession has illustrated how the NHS and its subsequent development differentially affected them. Although the hospital consultants have been the more power-ful group during this time in terms of impact upon health policy and in terms of their earnings, the GPs witnessed a significant revival in these two areas with the creation of their Royal College and the introduction of the Doctor's Charter. The 1980s was a difficult decade for both GPs and hospital consultants as managerialism entered the hospital sector and GPs were subjected to the limited prescribing list. However, while hospital consultants were subjected to indirect chal-lenges, GPs were faced with both indirect and direct challenges to their position. Indirectly, the transformation of the Family Prac-titioner Committees into Family Health Service Authorities (FHSA) sought to reconstitute this agency from a payroll office into a man-agerial authority to which GPs would be accountable (Warwicker, 1998). However, the new GP contract in 1990 represented a direct challenge to this section of the medical profession. This episode was significant because the government felt able to impose a health policy directly upon a section of the medical profession that was bitterly opposed to its introduction. By singling out GPs the government was to a certain extent illustrating that it felt able to challenge them directly while it was still using indirect methods upon hospital consultants, illustrating that Bevan's assessment of consult-ants' dominant position within the medical profession was still true 40 years on.

If one was to draw a balance sheet for the two sections of the medical profession by the end of 1990, on the eve of the introduction of the market reforms one would have to conclude that at both the micro and macro levels hospital consultants were dominant over GPs within the health service. At the micro level GPs were still com-plaining that discharge summaries either were never sent or they experienced lengthy delays in their receipt from hospital consultants. GPs had only a limited access to hospital-based diagnostic services, and outreach clinics run by hospital consultants in GP surgeries were still rare. GPs felt impotent to change these features and hospital consultants did not feel the need to modify their work practices to suit GPs. At the individual GP and hospital consultant level it was the hospital consultant who held sway over the service and the GPs had few if any levers by which to influence what went on within the hospital sector (Mahmood, 2001). At the macro level it was also clear that although the medical profession had lost influence as a whole it was the GPs who were left particularly weakened after the imposition of a controlling contract upon them in 1990. In contrast, hospital consultants had been able largely to neutralize assaults such as the introduction of general management into their sector. Thus, within a general landscape of a medical profession under assault it is the hospital consultants who were the first among equals as it entered the final decade of the twentieth century. The 1990s was to be a decade of enormous health sector reform in England.

AN INTERNAL MARKET FOR THE NHS

The 1991 NHS reforms have to be looked at in detail both in terms of the policies themselves and their political context. The reforms resulted from yet another perceived NHS funding 'crisis', but they can also be seen in the context of a long line of reforms to the service and the rising tide of managerialism. For the successful implementation of the 1991 NHS reforms, the government needed the management foundations that had been recommended by Griffiths in the 1980s (Mark and Scott, 1992), although it would be naive to suggest that this was all part of an elaborate preconceived plan. Rather, it represented the logic of hindsight and not foresight on the part of the government (Harrison, 1994, p. 149). The Griffiths reforms resulted in the creation of a clear management structure, both in district health authorities (DHAs) and the hospital sector, that could be charged with implementing this new and far more radical programme of reform. Indeed, the renewed importance of health service management was illustrated by the fact that the numbers of managers rose from just over 6,000 in 1989/90 to well over 20,000 in 1992/93 (Ham, 1997).

Market principles were particularly attractive to the Thatcher administration as they potentially provided a mechanism by which to challenge the professions, whom it saw as a largely unaccountable group (Light, 2001). Towards the end of the 1980s there was much media comment on a funding crisis in the NHS. Pictures and stories of patients, particularly children, suffering because of a perceived inadequately funded NHS finally forced the government to act (Butler,

1993). The prime minister announced in January 1988 that a working group had been set up to carry out a review of the service. This response represented the latest in a long line of administrative solutions to what were seen largely as resource problems within the service.

The 1989 White Paper *Working for Patients* (Department of Health, 1989g) was not the culmination of extensive consultations with the various NHS stakeholders or a lengthy royal commission; instead it resembled the ministerially driven Griffiths Inquiry of 1983. However, unlike the Griffiths Inquiry the prime ministerial review of the NHS that began its work in 1988 was an internal government affair. The review committee was made up of a small group of Department of Health officials, the chancellor and cabinet staff with the inclusion of some advisers and was chaired by the then prime minister, Margaret Thatcher. The blueprint for the largest reorganization of the NHS since its inception was completed within a year, it consisted of closed meetings, and it did not engage in formal consultations with the usual interest groups (Paton, 1990).

The working party decided to maintain the original principle of an NHS mainly funded from general taxation and it also decided that developing an internal market within the service would be the best way of restructuring the NHS in an effort to make it more efficient. The internal market idea for the NHS was loosely based on the North American thoughts expressed in Professor Enthoven's *Reflections on the Management of the NHS* (1985). However, when the White Paper and subsequently the various working papers were published the government had made many changes and significant additions to Enthoven's original ideas for the NHS. Creating autonomous hospital trusts and the development of budget-holding GPs were not advocated in Enthoven's 1985 reflections.

The central feature of the NHS reforms was the creation of an internal market that would cast the DHAs as buyers, and the independent hospital trusts as sellers, of health services. A somewhat late addition to this internal market structure were the GPs, who if they satisfied certain criteria on list sizes could become responsible for their own budgets from which they would purchase some of their patients' health care services. This new structure would mean that DHAs would no longer be responsible for managing and funding their district's health services; instead they would be responsible only for purchasing what they considered to be the necessary services for their resident population. The internal market's aim was that the various hospital trusts would compete for business with each other and with the private health care sector. The purchasers, in the form of DHAs and budget-holding GPs, would be responsible for buying the appropriate level of services for their patients from providers that offered the best deals in terms of price and quality. The government explained that these structural changes would improve organization of the service in a number of ways. There would be an improvement in the management of resources as money would begin to follow patients to efficient providers; clinicians would be more accountable for the resources they used; DHAs could concentrate solely on their new task of measuring their population's health care needs; and the new self-governing hospital trusts would benefit as they responded to the pressures of competition (Butler, 1993).

During 1989 and much of 1990 the government was stressing the market principles upon which the new NHS was to be based and was keen to use the commercial language of marketing, prices, contracts, buyers and sellers. However, by the end of 1990 the government was seeking to take away the commercial edge of their proposed reforms. In its bid to dampen any public fears concerning the privatization of the NHS, the official language changed: 'buyers' were first transformed into 'purchasers' and later 'commissioners'; 'sellers' became 'providers'; and 'marketing' was termed 'needs assessment'.

Along with the language change there was also to be a change in government strategy. The first year of the so-called market that came into operation on 1 April 1991 was to be a period of 'steady state'. Thus, it was becoming clear that the Conservative government's internal market was to be a market in name only. It is also important to comment upon the environment upon which the market reforms were being implemented. Even if the government had wanted to unleash the full power of competition upon the service, it still had the existing countervailing powers of the medical profession and the accumulated set of understandings that exist within the health care context to contend with (Light, 2001). Although the government and the countervailing powers tempered the free market thrust of the reforms, it would be mistaken to think that this structural transformation did not represent immense change for the NHS and for all those working within it. Light (2001) has argued that the implementation of the 1991 market reforms into the NHS

> *largely failed, yet profoundly changed power relations, the nature of the medical profession, the organisational matrix of health care, and its culture.* (p. 1168)

As far as primary care was concerned, the reforms offered GPs the opportunity to become directly involved in purchasing health services for their patients. These new structures potentially represented a framework for the greater regulation of hospital doctors. On the one hand hospital managers would attempt to control the work of their hospital consultants so that it reflected the trusts' corporate goals rather than the sometimes perceived esoteric interests of consultants, and on the other they would have GPs specifying in contracts, by way of quality standards, how their patients should be treated. Prior to the 1991 NHS reforms hospital consultants alone were responsible for defining the quality of their work, but in the new NHS medical audit and contract specifications could potentially regulate their work and in this way the 1991 reforms succeeded in linking quality with regulation.

The issue of quality has been a prominent feature of many of the policy initiatives within the public services, emerging in the NHS during the 1980s. For example, performance indicators were developed in 1982 for regional health authorities and DHAs (Ham, 1985). Standard setting continued in the 1990s with the introduction of the Patients' Charter and hospital league tables (Department of Health, 1991). The evidence of contracting in the NHS indicates that purchasers specified various quality standards and although all purchasers considered cost as their top priority, hospital trusts perceived quality as being the second priority of fundholding practices (Paton, 1998). However, the difficulty of measuring clinical quality, due to the lack of data, resulted in a tendency to concentrate on process-type issues such as waiting times, patient satisfaction, and the requirement for clinicians to undertake medical audit (Ham, 1997). Although instruments such as medical audit and contract specifications could potentially be used to regulate hospital consultants, it is open to question to what extent they were so used in practice. The introduction of the contracting process was a crucial plank of the reforms and it was to be the vehicle by which fundholding GPs could specify the volume, price and quality of the health services they would purchase for their patients. The regulation of quality through the contracting process in the internal market was the latest illustration of the introduction of regulatory devices for performance and standards in the hospital sector.

GPs AS PURCHASERS

Certain commentators considered the advent of GP fundholding as the 'wild card' within the whole pack of the 1991 NHS reforms

(Glennerster, Matsaganis, Owens and Hancock, 1993; 1994). However, the creation of GP fundholders fitted well within this set of
reforms whose thrust was particularly aimed at controlling hospital consultants (Light, 2001). It was thought that by giving
certain GP practices the ability to purchase a range of health services
directly they would be able to make hospital consultants more
responsive (Light, 2001). GPs were initially timid in volunteering
for this scheme – only 7 per cent of them entered it in January
1991 (Ham, 1997) and the medical profession, in the form of the
BMA, was firmly opposed to the development of fundholding
within general practice. However, with time the scheme became
increasingly popular and by 1997 nearly 50 per cent of GPs
were part of fundholding practices covering over half of the
GP-registered population (Ham, 1997). By this time even the BMA
had to drop its opposition to the scheme as its members were
voting with their feet, thereby making the association's opposition
untenable.

For many GPs the fundholding scheme offered them the opportunities that many of them had been waiting for. Although general
practice had experienced something of a revival in the 1960s and
1970s, as the previous section illustrated the professional division in
terms of status still existed between the two branches of medicine.
GP fundholding represented a way for GPs to shift the balance
of power within the medical profession towards general practice.
Research carried out by Glennerster and his colleagues (1993) into
the GP fundholding scheme reported that one of the main reasons
that GPs gave for joining the scheme in the first wave was a desire to
shake up the hospital sector so as to improve the service their
patients received. They reported dissatisfaction in the lengthy waiting times and what they perceived as generally unhelpful hospital
consultants. A majority of GPs also felt that fundholding would
allow them to develop the services they could offer to their patients
within primary care. They wanted to provide a greater range of on-
site services such as physiotherapy and counselling. Later waves of
fundholders had been impressed by the perceived improvements
their earlier wave colleagues had received. GPs reported joining the
scheme in later waves because they had seen how fundholders were
able to make the hospital sector more responsive. Others joined the
scheme because they had been dissatisfied with their lack of influence upon their health authority's purchasing decisions and felt that
fundholding would give them the chance to make the changes in the
contracts they felt were necessary.

As far as the hospital sector was concerned Glennerster *et al.* (1993) reported that hospital managers and consultants were not taking first-wave fundholders very seriously, possibly due to their low numbers. Those working in the hospital sector did not properly understand the GP fundholding scheme and were slow to respond to fundholders' requests. GP fundholders annoyed both hospital and health authority managers as they made it increasingly clear that there were changes they wanted to make to the previous health authorities' contracts. The hospital managers soon realized that they would have to negotiate with their new GP purchasers or else face losing some of their contracts. An improvement in hospital laboratory services was an early target for first-wave fundholders, as they particularly wanted to see these services speeded up and there were private laboratory services that GPs could contract with if their local hospital was unwilling to respond to their demands. Glennerster and his colleagues (1993) found numerous examples of hospitals responding to GP fundholders' demands as these GPs threatened to move a contract from an initially unresponsive hospital. The researchers reported upon other important cultural shifts, citing the example of one fundholding GP's astonished comments regarding the fact that he was having regular meetings with the hospital consultants:

> *No consultant has ever talked to me about what I might think of his service or any general problems we might have in twenty years of professional life.* (Glennerster, Matsaganis, Owens and Hancock, 1993, p. 93)

This study of GP fundholding illustrated how fundholders were 'flexing their purchasing muscle' in order to make hospitals, and particularly hospital consultants, more responsive. Most of the quality specifications that the fundholders made were not to do with clinical quality but instead were concerned with process-type issues such as the content and speed of discharge summaries and waiting times for a first outpatient consultation. As well as being able to challenge secondary care services in the ways described above, GP fundholders began to examine whether they could relocate certain hospital services into their practices. Their ability to manage their own budget meant that instead of paying for hospital physiotherapy services, for example, they could use their funds to employ a physiotherapist to see patients in the GP surgery. It is important to realize that even as the purchasing that GP fundholders could undertake expanded into community health services they were still only responsible for contracting 20 per cent of hospital and community services, the remaining 80 per cent of services being managed by their local health authority (Ham, 1997). This fact meant that fundholders could be flexible purchasers, able to move certain contracts between providers without causing a hospital trust to go out of business – something a health authority risked if it moved its much larger contracts in any major way. This meant that fundholding GPs were able to exert pressure on hospitals to increase their micro efficiency and quality.

The changes that fundholders managed to make, although small, were succeeding in altering the balance of power between themselves and hospital consultants. Other research into the impact of GP-led commissioning schemes reported on improved collaboration among GPs (Smith, Regen, Shapiro and Baines, 2000), a factor that would later be extended with the creation of PCGs (Baeza and Campbell, 2001 and Baeza, 2004). The GP population had traditionally been a rather fragmented group, so any initiatives that would increase the level of collaboration among them would be likely to increase their influence within the health care system.

Fundholding was not the only means by which GPs were beginning to contribute to what the provision of health services for their patients should be. Most of the remaining 50 per cent of the non-fundholding GP population was becoming involved in the purchasing process by engaging in a range of schemes such as locality purchasing and practice-sensitive purchasing (Ham, 1997). One study into an alternative way that GPs were inputting into a health authority's contracting process reported that 75 per cent of the quality targets and 55 per cent of the service developments planned for the individual hospital directorates had come largely from the GPs (Graffy and Williams, 1994). Although in the main these types of arrangements did not generally give GPs as much influence as the fundholding scheme, they contributed to the increasing importance GPs were having in the health care system as a whole.

Commentators have argued that one of the main results of the 1991 reforms was a shift in the balance of power within the service (Klein, 1995; Ham, 1997). The overall power shift was from a service that had largely been supply-led to one that would have a greater potential to be purchaser-led. This argument would suggest that the balance of power would swing from consultants who were now employed by providers to those GPs who had decided to become purchasers within GP fundholding practices, and other non-fundholding GPs who were also engaged in joint purchasing with health authorities to varying extents. A review of the development of the GP fundholding scheme by Dixon and Glennerster (1995) argued that

> *Fundholders are challenging the traditional interface of primary and secondary care and offering more services in house. Significant improvements in access to and the process of care have been secured by some fundholders. Giving budgets to general practitioners has been associated with a noticeable change in their relationship with hospital consultants.* (p. 729)

Flynn (1992) attributed the importance of fundholding GPs to the fact that they are part of the medical profession and it is this fact that enabled them to speak with authority when demanding quality standards from health care providers. North (1998) also found in her research that when GPs and hospital consultants met, a shared professional culture could be observed. A medically qualified informant stated to her that *'one of the less attractive characteristics of medics is that they rarely will give the same degree of credence to a non-medic . . .'* (p. 11). McKee and Clarke (1995) suggested that the creation of fundholding GPs would enable them to establish a more equitable relationship between the surgery and the hospital. Although the new structures developed by the NHS reforms did potentially create an environment where such a shift in power could occur, the real interest lies in how and to what extent these potentials would be realized at a local level where the environment is much more complex. Before going on to consider the changes the 1997 Labour government were to introduce into the NHS it is worth reflecting on the actual impact of the Conservatives' NHS reform programme.

THE IMPACT OF REFORM

The 1991 package of NHS reforms tended to favour primary care and GPs rather than the hospital sector and hospital consultants (Klein, 1995). Although the NPM-style policies in the 1980s had been largely ineffective in controlling the medical profession, they did have a cumulative impact on it by suggesting to people inside and outside the NHS that the time was right for change. The mere fact that health service reform was discussed and then introduced suggests that the medical profession had lost some of its influence by being unable to stifle reform. The culture had changed and it was now legitimate to question the medical profession; and the profession had to be ready to defend itself, which in certain areas it did, thus showing that it still retained some of its power. Not only was the 1991 package of reforms far-reaching and potentially threatening to the profession, it was also being implemented upon a weakened medical profession. As a result of some key environmental changes that had occurred during the intervening years, the medical profession in the 1990s was in a much weaker position than it had been in the 1940s and the concessions it could gain from governments were limited. It may be that the so-called 'wild card' in the NHS reforms represented the largest threat to hospital consultants, that is, the introduction of general practitioner fundholding. Moreover, the fact that a large proportion of GPs became fundholders against the opinion of many of the profession's organizations suggests that there was a certain amount of disunity within the medical profession.

The 1990s therefore represented a time when GPs became the key players within the NHS. Not only were GPs becoming more influential in deciding the type and form of hospital services that should be provided for their patients, they were also becoming responsible for actually providing more services within primary care. A 'primary care-led NHS' was becoming a much used phrase in NHS circles. Ham (1997) pointed to four examples of the move towards this type of NHS: an increase in the shared care of patients with chronic diseases such as asthma and diabetes; hospital consultants holding more of their clinics in GP surgeries; GP practices undertaking a wider range of diagnostic tests in-house; and GPs increasingly employing a wider range of staff such as physiotherapists and counsellors, allowing them to offer a range of in-house services to their patients. Fundholding GPs were often in the vanguard of these developments within primary care as has already been illustrated. Furthermore, government policy under the Conservative administration tended to favour GP fundholders. When the management costs within the NHS were rising, it was only GP fundholding practices that were exempt from any such cuts (Ham, 1997). However, as well as gaining more influence within the NHS, GPs themselves were also becoming increasingly managed. The closer management of GPs had begun in 1990 with the introduction of the new contract (Department of Health, 1989a). This continued throughout the 1990s as Family Health Service Authorities (FHSAs) merged with already merged DHAs to become large unitary health authorities. The new health authorities that were responsible for managing GPs' performance were in a much better state to carry out the management function than their FHSA predecessors. So it can be seen that one of the drawbacks for GPs of their increasing influence was that they were becoming subjected to a greater degree of management inspection by the new health authorities.

Although it is easy to overstate the impact of the 1991 reforms, it would be equally wrong to suggest that they had little effect upon the NHS and the professionals who work within it. There are various examples of micro changes that individually could be seen as somewhat insignificant when an overall review of the reforms is undertaken. It is these small changes within the service coupled with other wider changes in society and the medical profession that may have profound implications upon the intraprofessional relations of hospital consultants and GPs.

The success of the Labour party at the 1997 general election was to herald yet another period of reform for the NHS.

A NEW NHS?

Various commentators have argued that the competitive thrust of the 1991 reforms had largely disappeared by 1995/96 and the themes of partnership and co-operation were being promoted (Light, 2001; Flynn and Williams, 1997). It is in this light that the first set of NHS reforms that the incoming New Labour government implemented has to be seen. Some observers have judged these reforms to be a continuation of the previous Conservative reforms in a new guise (Light, 2001). Although there are discernable differences between the 1991 and the first post-1997 set of reforms, there has also been much continuity (particularly most recently) and many of the differences are more about style than substance (Surrender and Fitzpatrick, 1999). In certain respects the Labour government's reforms make many of the measures that were introduced in 1991 more explicit. For example in the 1991 reforms the documents relating to medical audit avoided stating that the scheme would be compulsory, but the 1999 reforms by contrast are quite clear that medical audit will be mandatory within both secondary and primary care.

The New Labour government's first NHS reforms that were largely implemented in 1999 were broadly based upon the 1997 Department of Health White Paper *The New NHS: Modern, Dependable*. This document made it clear that it did not plan to reverse the whole raft of structural changes that had been implemented in 1991; indeed it begins by stating that '*These changes will build on what has worked, but discard what has failed* (Department of Health, 1997, para 1.3). In the new government's considered opinion the commissioner/ provider split had worked but the internal market had failed and it proposed to

> . . . *go with the grain of recent efforts by NHS staff to overcome the obstacles of the internal market. Increasingly those working in primary care, NHS trusts, and health authorities have tried to move away from outright competition towards a more collaborative approach.* (Department of Health, 1997, para. 2.2)

Again, this paragraph recognizes that real competition had long ceased to exist in the NHS, if indeed it ever had existed – an observation that has been made by other research (Flynn, Williams and Pickard, 1996). The new set of reforms sought to instil a culture of collaboration both within the health service and between the NHS and other agencies such as local authorities and social services.

The new reforms retained trust status for hospitals but abolished annual contracts in favour of three- to five-year funding agreements. In a similar way to the 1991 reforms, many of those of 1999 were portrayed as necessary developments that would improve the quality of health care within the NHS. In fact a whole separate document was devoted to these new quality measures (Department of Health, 1998), which proposed a new set of quality improvement initiatives that would operate at both national and local levels. National standards for managing various diseases in the form of National Service Frameworks (NSFs) have been published, which contain specific timetabled targets for both secondary and primary care (see for example the NSF for coronary heart disease, Department of Health, 2000b). The development of NSFs is significant as it replaces the flexibility of local standards – which were considered sufficient in the 1991 reforms – with national norms. Centrally set standards such as NSFs could potentially damage the local autonomy that is the foundation of doctors' micro power (Pollitt, 1993a).

Two new national organizations have been created under the new administration. The National Institute for Clinical Excellence (NICE) is responsible for issuing evidence-based guidelines on both clinical procedures and drugs. The second body, initially the Commission for Health Improvement (CHI) and now the Healthcare Commission, is responsible for monitoring the quality of health service organizations via a rolling programme of visits to both secondary and primary care organizations.

At a local level a new system of clinical governance was implemented that has given trust chief executives a responsibility for the quality of their services to match their financial responsibilities. Clinical governance incorporates various measures such as evidence-based practice, medical audit, risk management, professional development and systems to manage poor performance. Although some of the mechanisms contained within clinical governance are not new, they have been given a greater emphasis by this new initiative. Within primary care, clinical governance represents a particular challenge, as many of these measures have not been widely implemented in this sector in the past. A central aim of the clinical governance framework was to make groups of professionals accountable for each other's performance. This represents a move from individual responsibility for quality of practice to a collective one (Allen, 2000). Table 2.1 summarizes the change in emphasis that these policies have collectively made upon health professionals in general and hospital clinicians in particular.

As far as primary care is concerned, the theme of continuity and change was repeated. The new administration abolished the GP fundholding scheme and replaced this voluntary scheme with the compulsory arrangements of primary care groups. PCGs have now become primary care trusts that are responsible for purchasing all their resident population's health services and are also the providers of primary and community health services. These new primary health structures can be seen to have many similarities with the Conservative government's GP fundholding scheme that had already established a number of GP total purchasing pilots where GPs were being allowed to contract for the full range of health and community services for their patients. The new structures for primary care are set to continue the trend of giving GPs a leading role within the NHS, a message that was made clear in the government's White Paper (Department of Health, 1989g):

> *The family doctor or community nurse is often the first port of call . . . They understand patients' needs and they deliver most*

Table 2.1   A shift in emphasis

Individual	→	*corporate* thinking
Professional	→	*multiple* accountability
Partial	→	*full* participation
Improvement	→	*and* assurance
Local	→	*and* national

local services. That is why they will be in the driving seat in shaping local health services in the future. (para. 5.1)

It is clear from the above quote that the Labour government, like its Conservative predecessor, wanted to continue to endow primary care and those working within it with the necessary powers to enable them to commission and provide the health services that they assess their local population to need. The White Paper continues to recognize the improvements that fundholding GPs had achieved and envisages the new primary care organizations as extending these benefits to the whole population:

> . . . *many innovative GPs and their fund managers have used the fundholding scheme to sharpen the responsiveness of some hospital services and to extend the range of services available in their own surgeries* . . . *Primary Care Groups will extend to all patients the benefits but not the disadvantages, of fundholding. By virtue of their size and financial leverage, they will have far greater ability to shape local services around patients' needs.* (Paras. 5.5 and 5.18)

The message from the Labour administration is thus clear: its intentions for primary care are to strengthen its ability both to commission *and* provide health and community services.

Taken as a whole, this package of health service reforms indicated that primary care's favoured position within the NHS was set to continue under the Labour administration, and Department of Health documents such as *Shifting the Balance of Power within the NHS* (2001c) made this an explicit policy. However, as has happened in the past, GPs' continued prominence within the health care arena comes at the cost of becoming ever more managerially controlled. Within PCTs, GPs will be more closely managed by both managers and fellow GPs. Studies have reported the fact that PCGs were more willing than health authorities to tackle issues regarding the poor performance of GPs (Baeza and Campbell, 2001 and Baeza, 2004). It is likely that the 'elite' GPs within PCTs will be in a position to manage other 'rank and file' GPs. However, within PCTs GPs and other clinicians will become increasingly managed by central PCT managers as their previous PCG influence declines (Dowling, Wilkin and Smith, 2003). The creation of the new primary care organizations led Klein and Maynard (1998) to suggest that

> *The attractions for government of creating a situation in which general practitioners improve resource use by controlling their*

colleagues are self-evident. The attractions for independent con-
tractor general practitioners are less apparent and they may not
comply. Indeed, the long-term implication may be that ministers
expect general practitioners to become salaried employees. (Klein
and Maynard, 1998, 5).

The increasing popularity of personal medical services may soon
make the salaried GP the norm in the NHS.

BACK TO THE FUTURE?

New Labour's appetite for health service reform was not satisfied in
its first term and continued into its second when the government
ushered in a whole new raft of NHS reforms and a second NHS plan
(Department of Health, 2004b). If the first NHS plan (Department
of Health, 2000a) was a mixture of continuity and change the latest
set of reforms have striking similarities to those of 1990. By April
2005, foundation hospitals had been created; payment by results and
patient choice were introduced; individual GP practices were now
able to apply to their PCT to allow them to commission services; and
new more regulatory contracts had been negotiated with hospital
consultants and GPs. These reforms have been accompanied by the
Labour government's large injection of spending into the NHS,
which will have increased from 6.8 per cent of gross domestic product in 1997 to 9.4 per cent in 2007–8, bringing UK health spending
in line with the European average (Stevens, 2004). Tony Blair has
insisted that the *quid pro quo* for this extra NHS expenditure is
that the service undergoes a process of 'modernization', New
Labour's preferred term for NPM-type public service reform. These
'new' NHS reforms are perhaps recognition that their first set of
reforms has not had the positive impact upon the service that they
had hoped for.

Hospitals that gain three stars from the Healthcare Commission
can apply for foundation status, which in theory will free them from
the control of the Department of Health, though they remain within
the NHS (Department of Health, 2002a). Many of the freedoms
offered to foundation hospitals closely resemble those that were first
promised to hospital trusts in the 1990 reforms, although there are
also differences which may mean that the twenty-first-century freedoms are not a chimera like those of the early 1990s. The foundation
hospitals will have a local mandate as their local population will

elect and form part of the hospitals' boards of governors. In order to avoid the accusation of inequity between foundation and non-foundation hospitals the government has stated that it envisages all hospitals achieving foundation status by 2008 (Department of Health, 2004b). If this occurs this policy may reinvigorate the hospital sector, particularly acute teaching hospitals, and make collaboration and integration with primary care more difficult (Walshe, 2003).

Although the internal market was formally abolished by the incoming Labour government in 1997 it is making a reappearance with government initiatives such as payment by results for hospital trusts (Department of Health, 2002b) and giving patients a degree of choice of where to have certain procedures performed (Department of Health, 2003a). Closely connected to these policies is practice-based commissioning, which from April 2005 has allowed individual GP practices to obtain indicative commissioning budgets from their host PCTs (Department of Health, 2004a). This may be an attempt by the government to re-energize general practices and provide them with incentives to engage with their PCTs by becoming involved in deciding what services hospitals will provide and in what manner they should be provided (Lewis, 2004). This package of policies has a definite 'retro' feel as together they seem to reintroduce many of the reforms that were first instigated in 1991: trust status for hospitals; a limited NHS internal market; and a form of GP fundholding.

After protracted negotiations (particularly in the case of hospital consultants) both GPs and hospital consultants have agreed on new contracts (Department of Health 2003b and 2004c). In the case of hospital consultants the new contract will mean greater accountability through job plans, although the degree to which these job plans allow managers to regulate hospital consultants' duties remains to be seen. The new contract makes consultants' commitment to the NHS stronger, particularly in their first seven years. The closed and almost incestuous system of distinction awards, that Bevan used to buy hospital consultant support for the creation of the NHS, will be abolished and replaced by the clinical excellence award scheme, which promises to be transparent, fair and based on clear evidence. In return for this new more regulatory contract hospital consultants will receive modest increases in their salary. The new GP contract allows GPs to opt out of providing certain services such as 24-hour care or indeed provide 'enhanced services' such as offering minor surgery. As well as being able to tailor the services that GPs offer the

NHS they will be able to earn around a third more. In return for these advantages GPs will have to provide services of a prescribed quality. Other clinicians such as nurses and therapists have also undergone national job evaluations and local job redesigns that are aimed at breaking down interprofessional demarcations and increase and expand multidisciplinary working in both secondary and primary care. Only time will tell what impact this large and varied package of reforms will have on the intraprofessional relations of GPs and hospital consultants, but it seems clear that primary care will continue to be centre-stage in the new NHS.

3

THE POLITICS OF THE MEDICAL PROFESSION

INTRODUCTION

This chapter will examine the issue of power within both the policy process and the medical profession. First, various approaches to power within the health policy process will be briefly considered and their strengths and weaknesses assessed. The medical profession itself will then be examined and the nature of its dominance within the health care system discussed. It will be suggested that the profession has been able to establish a professional dominance within the British National Health System (NHS) that has been guarded against external threats. This chapter will argue that although the medical profession has come under threat from various sources its relative power within the health care system has remained largely intact. Alford's (1975) structural approach to power and his framework of structural interests in relation to health policy will then be examined in more detail. Finally, this structural-interests approach will be used to carry out an analysis of contemporary health policy in order to illustrate its utility for the aims of this study.

DEFINING POWER

Before one can begin to study and analyse the medical profession, its power and the possible changes in the power relations within the profession, it is first important to consider the concept of power within the policy process and the different perspectives there are upon it. This follows the approach first developed by Ham in his first edition of his book *Health Policy in Britain* (Ham, 1982). Ham argued that it is crucial to analyse the distribution of power in health systems in order properly to understand the policy process. To do this one must consider the literature on political theory and the three broad theoretical approaches that will be considered, mirroring Ham's approach, are:

- Pluralist and neo-pluralist approaches
- Marxist and neo-Marxist approaches
- Structuralist or elite theory approaches

PLURALIST APPROACHES

The classical pluralist takes the view that the policy arena is influenced by different groups and that no one group is dominant, rather the relative influence of a group will depend on the situation. The view that power is shared ensures that health policy is determined by the outcome of negotiations between the various pressure groups (Dahl, 1961). This pressure group perspective can be a useful framework for policy analysis as it can be used to concentrate on the micro relations between the various players. However, it is flawed in so far as it ignores the relative power of the various stakeholders by suggesting that no one group is dominant. Pluralists argue that power is shared among the different pressure groups and policy decisions will be essentially democratic in nature, as they will reflect the particular balance of power of these interest groups. However, when applied to health policy, this ignores the dominance of the medical profession. This approach therefore offers no explanations as to why and how the medical profession holds such a dominant position within the health service. There are marked disparities in the influence of the various groups on the health policy-making process; it is these disparities that are of great importance and worthy of further analysis.

Neo-pluralists (Lindblom, 1977) have refined the position of the earlier classical pluralists by recognizing that some groups are more influential than others. They highlight the powerful position of large corporations and the state within the policy process. However, neo-pluralists still argue that although some groups have privileged positions, the policy process is still characterized by negotiation and the need for a balance to be struck between the various players. They also point to the fact that much of the bargaining process is not carried out in arenas such as parliament but discussions occur among networks made up of senior officials. In the case of health policy, it would be officials from the Department of Health, senior health authority managers and various professional representatives who would make up these networks which, in the neo-pluralists' view, help to avoid major conflicts from occurring. The pluralist and neo-pluralist views are useful in as much as they point out the importance of different interest groups within the policy process. However, although neo-pluralists recognize that some of the players in the policy-making arena hold privileged and powerful positions they fail to take into account the structural foundations of these. These power differentials will impact on policy negotiations and mean that policy decisions are not as unpredictable and democratic as neo-pluralist theory might suggest.

MARXIST APPROACHES

Marxist analysts argue that medicine is useful to capitalism as a legitimizing force, by defining ill health as an individualistic disease-based model and thus ignoring the structural causes of ill health. This helps to maintain the dominant position of the bourgeoisie and allows it to appear to care about the working class (Navarro, 1976). Other Marxist commentators, such as Larkin (1983) have argued that medicine commands the privileged position it does from the state because it fulfils the needs of capital by keeping the workforce healthy and assisting in the reproduction of labour, thus allowing for the accumulation of capital. Marxists argue that expenditure within the health service can also be explained by their class analysis. That is to say that services directed at the mentally ill and elderly are of low priority because these groups are not economically product-ive and cannot therefore contribute to a capitalist society. Thus, the state directs its limited resources to the capitalist project by maintain-ing a healthy workforce and helping to reproduce future workers (O'Connor, 1973; Gough, 1979).

Although the legitimating function of health care that Marxists point to is convincing, their production function argument is sim-plistic, ignoring how largely ineffective medicine has been in this area. McKeown (1979) has argued that the medical interventions can account for only minor achievements in the rise of the popula-tion's health; better nutrition and environmental hygiene have had the largest impacts on the nation's health. If the medical profession concentrated on the needs of capital and its need for a healthy workforce it would focus on common illnesses and disorders as well as on health promotion and illness prevention. However, it is evident that the reverse is true – the medical profession values research into rare and interesting disorders and curing acute illnesses; in other words it fulfils its own needs rather than directly those of capital. Nevertheless, it should be remembered that it is the state that grants the profession the privileged position it has and so it is to the profession's advantage to assist the state as its patron and sponsor. However, a rigid Marxist analysis makes the mistake of oversimplifying what is a complex relationship between the state, society and the profession. Although on a macro level this perspective has explanatory value it is weak when one looks at the micro dynamics of policy formulation and implementation within the health service.

In terms of the distribution of power within the health sector, Navarro (1978) has argued that the medical profession does not in fact possess its own autonomy – he views the medical profession as being like all other groups of workers who are subject to the political and ideological hegemony of capital. This analysis is also simplistic, suggesting in a deterministic and functionalist way that all workers are slaves to capital without differentiating between them. The medical profession's power and autonomy within the health system cannot be denied and must be understood when considering health policy analysis. Although it would be wrong to argue that the medical profession has complete autonomy, of interest to this study is the profession's autonomy relative to others inside and outside of the health system and its relative internal autonomy; hence interprofessional and intraprofessional autonomy need to be analysed. Marxist theory takes a very broad view and by attempting to look at structures as being interconnected and historical in nature it overlooks the micro policy environment and the theory's explanatory value is restricted to an overview. This weakness means that it is an unsatisfactory theory for explaining the micro factors involved in health policy formulation and implementation, and thus remains a tool that is restricted to a macro analysis.

STRUCTURALIST APPROACHES

A structuralist approach to policy analysis helps to fill in many of the gaps left by the Marxist and pluralist perspectives. This approach has the advantage of recognizing the influence of structure on power relations and helps to explain how different structural arrangements give dominance to certain structural interests. The structuralist approach recognizes the value of the Marxist perspective by acknowledging the importance of economic and class differences. However, this theory maintains that the important divisions rest between the different structural interests. In common with the pluralist tradition it acknowledges that the policy process is influenced by different interest groups, but it argues that there are differences in power between these groups that are based on their structural interests. Pluralism sees policy making as occurring in an arena consisting of many different groups, which are not ordered in any particular way, which are voluntary and competitive and which negotiate and come to a balanced compromise. In contrast, structuralist approaches within elite theory such as neo-corporatism view the policy process as consisting of only a limited number of producer groups who are recognized by the state and granted representation in exchange for them recognizing certain state set parameters. Cawson (1982) argues that

> *Power in the corporate sector is not determined by resources, membership and publicity but is exercised within a context that is structurally given by the division of labour.* (p. 43)

Parliament has a rubber-stamping role in such a process, where the deals are struck between the favoured elite and are then promoted to their rank and file. In this sense Harrison (1994) states that

> *Corporatist relationships are between government and producer groups, that is, extra-parliamentary and managerialist in character.* (p. 147)

The British health policy process fits well into this framework, with the medical profession being a classic state-sponsored elite whose representatives such as the British Medical Association (BMA) and the royal colleges negotiate with senior officials in the relevant departments over policy decisions. Alford's (1975) structural interests framework also fits into elite theory and has certain similarities to the neo-corporatist approach. Alford argues that health policy is characterized by intense competition between the different elite groups. He makes an important differentiation between an 'interest group' and what he terms 'structural interests' and he defines the latter as

> *. . . those interests served or not served by the way they 'fit' into the basic logic and principles by which the institutions of a society*

operate ... These are interests which are more than potential interest groups which are merely waiting for the opportunity or the necessity of organizing to present demands or grievances to the appropriate authorities. (p. 14)

Alford's framework identifies three structural interests: dominant, challenging and repressed, which in his account of the New York City health system are represented respectively by the medical profession, health administrators and the community without health insurance. Before going on to examine Alford's theoretical framework in greater depth and how it will be used in this study it is important to consider the nature and basis of the medical profession's dominance. These are important discussions, as they will help inform Alford's theoretical framework that will be used to consider how the structural changes to the English health care system over the past 15 years have affected the relative dominance of the two branches of the medical profession.

MEDICAL DOMINANCE

After considering various definitions of power within the health policy process it is necessary to contextualize power within health care with particular reference to the medical profession. It is important to examine the medical profession's dominance within the health care arena and how it has managed to preserve this position.

When analysing the literature on the professions it is all too easy to become engulfed in a debate about which are the characteristics that define a profession and which occupations can be defined as professions and which are those that cannot. Trait theory, as the name suggests, was an attempt to classify a profession by the nature of its characteristics or its 'traits' (Millerson, 1964; Goode, 1960). This theory is highly problematic and lacks any explanatory value because it either attempts to list all the characteristics of a profession, thus allowing occupations such as electricians and plumbers to be included or else it is too specific, only including the classical professions such as medicine and the clergy. However, as the focus of this study is to analyse the intraprofessional relations of the medical profession I will not dwell on the question of 'what is a profession?' Rather, I will concentrate on examining how and why the medical profession possesses the power it does. Before taking a more detailed examination of the medical profession it is worth discussing the wider literature surrounding the professions as a whole and their place in society so as to put the medical profession within a broader context.

Functionalists such as Carr-Saunders and Wilson (1933) viewed the professions as a stabilizing force within society and as important maintainers of tradition. They described them as valuable conservative forces who

> ... *inherit, preserve and pass on a tradition* ... *they engender modes of life, habits of thought and standards of judgement which render them centres of resistance to crude forces which threaten steady and peaceful evolution* ... *The family, the church and the universities, certain associations of intellectuals, and above all the great professions, stand like rocks against which the waves raised by these forces beat in vain.* (p. 497)

Both functionalists and trait theorists tended to view the professions from the professionals' own rhetoric and values, rather than taking a critical outsider's view. These perspectives failed to look at what Johnson (1972) has described as '*the characteristics of a historically specific institutionalised form of its control*' (p. 27). In other words both the trait and functionalist approaches fail to examine the environment in which the professions exist. Environmental factors such as the social standing of a profession's clientele both in time and space would help explain why, for example, the prestige of a primary school teacher is (arguably) lower than that of the university lecturer. This form of analysis would also help to explain why the hospital consultant who receives professionally referred patients (that is, referred to the consultant by a GP) has a higher status than the GP who attends to the self-referring public (Calnan, 1981).

Johnson (1972) has argued that the professions that can produce what are seen as specialized products are able to achieve what he calls 'social distance' by creating a social and economic dependence on the part of the consumers of this specialized product. This kind of producer–consumer relationship has a certain level of indeterminacy: the higher the level of indeterminacy the more unbalanced will be the power relation between the two. It is important to note that this indeterminacy can be real or perceived, for example the technical nature of the clergy's work is not in itself complex and their status is instead derived from the perceived spiritual nature of their knowledge. As society's perceptions change then so the status of certain professions changes, helping to explain the decline in the status of the clergy within an increasingly secular society. However, a profession's status is not solely dependent on society's perceptions of their knowledge – a profession can gain power from other sources; the state can grant certain professions power. If we continue with the example of the clergy, the state allows the church certain influence in the policy-making process by giving some of them seats in the House of Lords, which could explain why the church has managed to maintain a disproportionately powerful place despite a fall in the importance of Christian values within British society. Society's own knowledge base is also important in determining the social distance a profession can achieve. As society's knowledge increases then so this social distance decreases, which is what has been experienced in the case of medicine in the past 20 or 30 years. It is these factors that are important and it is because of these that a profession cannot usefully be described as a set of qualities or an end state; instead, professionalism is historically specific (Freidson, 1994). Johnson (1972) describes the producer–consumer relationship in the following way:

> *The power relationship existing between practitioner and client may be such, then, as to enable the practitioner to increase the social distance and its own autonomy and control over practice by engaging in a process of 'mystification'. Uncertainty is not, therefore, entirely cognitive in origin but may be deliberately increased to serve manipulative or managerial ends.* (pp. 42–3)

Johnson (1972) argues that there are three types of producer–consumer relationship and these display varying balances of power between the two groups. Collegiate control is displayed when the producer has a high level of autonomy and is able to define the needs of the consumer and the manner in which these are supplied. This type of control needs the state's legitimacy: in the UK the state has given the medical profession a monopoly role as the supplier of health care and has allowed the profession to define illness, for example, by being able to provide patients with a doctor's certificate that has legal status. The deserving poor who used the voluntary hospitals in the nineteenth and early twentieth centuries would have been under this collegiate form of control, as it was the doctor who determined the needs of the patient and how these should be treated. A relationship of patronage is present when the consumer is able to define their own needs and the manner in which these needs are met. This would have been the situation for the upper classes in Britain in the nineteenth and early part of the twentieth centuries who retained the services of various professions including doctors and priests under a form of oligarchic patronage. Lastly, a mediative relationship lies somewhere between the previous two situations. In this type of relationship there is a third party who mediates between the producer and consumer. Medicine within the welfare state is supplied within a relationship of mediative control, and the state is the third party that intervenes and influences the type and manner of services that are available to its citizens. These different types of relationships will have particular consequences for a profession's autonomy; however, what is of more importance is how a profession functions under these different types of control. Although the majority of medicine in the UK is supplied under the state's mediation through the NHS, the medical profession has been successful in being able to define large parts of its work. In contrast, the teaching profession within the education system, which is also largely supplied in a similar way, has not been as successful in defining its work.

Johnson (1972) argues that the greater amount of homogeneity a profession displays the stronger it will tend to be. A profession that has a common outlook, a low degree of specialization and recruits from similar backgrounds will tend to be cohesive and therefore be more resistant to outside influences. In the nineteenth and early twentieth centuries the medical profession displayed many of these characteristics; however, throughout the twentieth century the profile of the profession has been changing. At the end of the twentieth century the medical profession displayed a high degree of specialization, a larger divergence in outlook and contained a greater number of recruits from varying social and economic backgrounds. The heterogeneous nature of the modern medical profession would tend to suggest that it was a weaker profession at the end of the twentieth century than at the beginning of it. Johnson (1972) has suggested that strong professional associations and registering bodies such as the BMA, the General Medical Council (GMC) and the royal colleges can foster cohesion in a profession; however, this ignores the differences between these organizations and the views of the rank and file members of the profession. A fragmented profession allows the consumer and the state to become more powerful participants within the profession–consumer–state relationship. However, these macro changes to the medical profession tell us nothing about the possible changes that have occurred *within* the profession. As the medical profession becomes more fragmented as a group it becomes more important to examine intraprofessional relations and study the possible impacts of these upon health policy.

INSIDE THE MEDICAL PROFESSION

The British medical profession's power was largely gained in the middle of the nineteenth century, when in 1858 the state granted it a market monopoly on doctoring. This was first strengthened and then weakened throughout the course of the twentieth century, as discussed in the previous chapter. There are many reasons why and how the medical profession has been able to gain such prominence. The vast literature on the professions contains various theories of how they amassed their power and how some professional groups have been more successful at this than others. Freidson's writings on the medical profession and his analysis of the roots of its power are important in this discussion (Freidson, 1970; 1986). Freidson (1970) makes it clear that there are political foundations to the medical profession's power; it is the state that sponsors the profession and grants it the autonomy it enjoys. The medical profession has successfully claimed that it possesses specialist knowledge and skills, which due to their complexity only fellow medical professionals are able to evaluate. It is these skills that the state requires within a system of health care and thus sponsors the profession and lends it its political support. It is not merely that the doctor makes claims of being an expert; it is the revered content, substance and mystical nature of their knowledge, be this real or implied, that is the important factor. As Freidson (1970) argues, it is

> *a process in which power and persuasive rhetoric are of greater importance than the objective character of knowledge, training and work.* (p. 83)

Turner (1987) has also suggested that it is the possession of such specialized and esoteric knowledge that has allowed the profession to make demands of autonomy upon the state in the area of health care, arguing that to obtain autonomy the profession's knowledge must

> *have a distinctive mystique which suggests that there is a certain professional attitude and competence which cannot be reduced merely to systematic and routinized knowledge.* (p. 136)

The state has often pointed to this specialized knowledge of the medical profession in order to justify granting it the autonomy it enjoys. The 1975 government-commissioned Merrison Report made this clear, stating that

> *It is the essence of a professional skill that it deals with matters unfamiliar to the layman, and it follows that only those in the*

*profession are in a position to judge many of the matters of stand-
ards of professional conduct which will be involved.* (p. 3)

In bureaucracies the expectation is that subordinates, due to their
hierarchical position in the organization, will obey officials. However,
this does not hold true when it comes to the NHS and the doctors
within it. As Freidson (1986) argues, professionals do not follow this
mode of work, instead they

> *. . . expect to be autonomous and self-directing, subject only to the
> constraints of competent knowledge and skill related to their task.
> They can accept advice, perhaps even orders, if it stems from
> someone of competence, but it is only competence, not official
> position as an administrative superior that is accepted as the
> source of effective authority over work.* (p. 159)

The essence of Freidson's observation is perfectly captured in the
remarks made by Mr Anthony Grabham, then chairman of the
BMA Council, when giving evidence to the House of Commons
Social Services Select Committee, 18 January 1984. He argued that:

> *If [a manager] took decisions which were harmful to our patients
> then we would not feel bound to co-operate with him [sic] in
> carrying out that decision.* (quoted in Harrison, 1999, p. 61)

Although Freidson tends somewhat to exaggerate the dominance
of the medical profession, it is true to say that the profession has
carved out a powerful niche within most health systems. This is what
Freidson (1986) describes as a 'shelter from the market', which gives
doctors freedoms and privileges that are unknown to professionals
in other organizations. He argues that the medical profession
achieves its market shelter by only allowing its tasks to be performed
by those who have been through a recognized course of higher education. In this respect it is important to note in terms of the differences between general practice and hospital medicine that it has been
hospital medicine that has had the greatest influence on medical
education in the UK (Hollingsworth, 1986). Although the majority
of Freidson's observations apply equally to the medical profession in
the UK, it is worth remembering that he was studying the medical
profession in the United States where health care is mainly private.
One of the consequences of a publicly funded system is that the
British medical profession will tend to have less economic autonomy
in terms of their NHS salaries, which are set by the state (although
this is not the case for the large number of doctors who also practise

in the private sector), and greater clinical autonomy then their US counterparts.

There are other important factors, which Freidson tends to overlook, such as financial restrictions and scientific limitations that constrain the medical profession's autonomy; these are important when investigating the power of the medical profession. It is possible to chart the medical profession's power by examining its relative success in maintaining its autonomy in the face of political and economic changes and challenges. However, setting these restrictions to one side, doctors have managed to create an almost unique position for themselves, not seen in other sectors. This is particularly true of the hospital doctor: the organizational structure of the hospital is such that the hospital consultant must be involved, either directly or indirectly, at all levels of a patient's treatment; his/her consent must be sought for treatments, medications, tests, admission, discharge, etc. The formal rules and procedures that are evident in other large bureaucracies and obeyed by other workers within the health sector do not apply to the medical profession; they have been able legitimately to avoid being controlled via bureaucratic norms. Furthermore, the medical profession has not only managed to control many aspects of its work, it has also been allowed to control medical education and training. This fact has allowed the profession to shape the future of medicine, favouring hospital medicine over primary care and acute care over chronic care (Wilding, 1982). The profession's choices often go against the notions of rational planning and the fact that the profession can do this is a reflection of its power. Using Lukes' (1974) ideas of power it could be said that the medical profession in general and hospital consultants in particular often display what he called 'third dimensional power', which he described as:

> . . . *prevent[ing] people, to whatever degree, from having grievances by shaping their perceptions, cognitions and preferences in such a way that they accept their role in the existing order of things, either because they can see or imagine no alternative to it, or because they can see it as natural and unchangeable, or because they value it as divinely ordained and beneficial?* (p. 24)

Freidson suggests that the medical profession's power can be gauged by the degree of autonomy and control it has over the technical character of its work (Freidson, 1970). Furthermore, he asserts that:

> *While no occupation can prevent employers, customers, clients and other workers from evaluating its work, only the profession*

has the recognized right to declare such 'outside' evaluation as illegitimate and intolerable. (Freidson, 1970:72)

The political nature of this power is clear: it is not that others such as employers or patients could not technically evaluate a doctor's work; the doctor's power rests on the fact that she or he can argue that such assessment is without basis and therefore irrelevant. Nevertheless, Freidson recognizes that the autonomy the medical profession enjoys is not absolute; rather it is dependent on the state and can thus undergo change. The self-regulation of the profession is state-sponsored and not an integral part of medicine, it is an outcome of the group's economic and political power, and this illustrates the profession's potential vulnerability to economic and political changes. The current debate over the self-regulation of health care professions in general and the medical profession in particular illus-trates this vulnerability (Smith, 1998; 1999). The medical profes-sion's autonomy is not unquestionable; it has to be defended and justified. Ultimately it is not the medical profession alone that will decide whether it maintains its privileged position and therein lies the profession's potential weakness. Salter (1998) has argued that the state can only agree to preserve the medical profession's autonomy if the profession retains the public's trust. However, the state can play and has played a part in influencing the public perception of the medical profession. By encouraging 'consumerism' within the NHS in the 1980s the Conservative government prompted the public to be more sceptical of the medical profession and thus allowed the gov-ernment to push through policies aimed at controlling it, showing that the state's role in this tripartite structure is of crucial importance.

Flynn (1992) has similarly argued that the medical profession's autonomy is relative and subject to change, stating that: '*Like all forms of human agency, medical autonomy is a relational attribute, having different manifestations and social-structural constraints*' (p. 24). Flynn is suggesting that as the three-way relations between the med-ical profession, the state and society change then so the profession's autonomy will change. Not only can medical autonomy alter but also it can change in a number of different ways. Flynn argues that medical autonomy is made up of various elements, these being eco-nomic, political and technical. The creation of the NHS may have weakened the medical profession's economic autonomy, as the majority of the profession was no longer free to determine the charges for their services, but by allowing themselves to be sponsored by the state they gained political autonomy.

Before moving on to examine the details of Alford's theoretical framework, which will be used in this study, it is worth briefly discussing the suggestion from certain analysts that the medical profession's power has been decreasing due to various structural changes in health care systems.

THE MEDICAL PROFESSION UNDER THREAT?

It has been argued that the medical profession is losing much of its power and autonomy due to increased outside scrutiny and cost-containment policies. However, these losses have not occurred equally across the profession; their impacts on hospital consultants and GPs have been different. The proponents of theories of the proletarianization of the medical profession (Derber, 1982) restrict their analysis to the macro level, failing to take account of the micro level of the health system where doctors are still responsible for directing resources according to their priorities as opposed to those of the government. So while the medical profession's autonomy may have decreased at the macro level, although not to the exaggerated levels that Derber (1982) has suggested, doctors have managed to retain most of their freedoms at the micro level, such as the hospital and the individual GP surgery. It should also be remembered that even the 1991 reforms explicitly restated the importance of doctors' self-regulation and their autonomy derived from this (Department of Health, 1997, p. 59; Department of Health, 1998, p. 46).

However, even if we accept that the medical profession as a corporate body has lost some of its professional power, at an individual level certain doctors have been more successful than others at maintaining their position. It is in the context of some sectors of the medical profession faring better than others, that Exworthy and Halford's (1999) argument of de-professionalization and re-professionalization is helpful. They suggest that while some sections of the medical profession have indeed been weakened or de-professionalized others have been re-professionalized leading to greater internal stratification within the profession, and one could examine the hospital consultants' and general practitioners' professional development in this way. Harrison (1999) has also suggested that power and autonomy have been redistributed within the profession rather than the profession actually losing it to other groups. Hoggett (1991) has argued that professionals themselves are being used to control fellow professionals; he suggests that there has been a change in approach:

> *. . . rather than attempt to strengthen 'management' in order to control 'professionals' the strategy shifts towards creating managers out of professionals . . . A new generation of unit managers begins to emerge who combine technical expertise with managerial competence.* (p. 254)

Dohler (1989) has suggested that the medical profession has lost much of its esteem and mystique, a factor that has and will continue to have an impact on the autonomy it enjoys. He points to the limitations of medicine and the decreasing gains it has made in its fight against illness and argues that advances in data-processing have increased the possibility for the economic standardization of a substantial part of medical practice. However, Dohler fails to recognize that while medicine cannot claim to have had an enormous impact on the population's ill health, in the past 50 years it has managed to keep developing so that new medical techniques such as organ transplants and *in vitro* fertilization are possible for people today. Although such advances have minimal gains for whole populations their promotion has allowed medicine to claim modern miracles that the public still holds in high esteem. Data-processing techniques have advanced in the past two decades but at the same time the profession has managed to restrict monitoring to the process functions of health care (issues such as lengths of stay and bed occupancy), leaving the 'art' of medicine as something that the profession has largely managed to control. This is particularly true in the UK, a fact that Dohler (1989) highlights, where tools such as performance indicators have been aimed mainly at managerial functions, allowing doctors largely to review and regulate their own work (Jost, 1992). However, in the United States, as Dohler (1989) points out, there is a plethora of reviews and checks that aim to standardize medical practice (Robinson and Stiener, 1998) and it is a matter of debate whether similar measures will be successfully introduced in the NHS. The importance of evidence-based medicine has increased in the past ten years and this represents a possible threat to the medical profession as it could potentially routinize health care and therefore restrict a doctor's clinical autonomy by making him/her a slave to evidence-based guidelines.

The literature on the professions that has been discussed helps explain how the medical profession has amassed its dominance within health care systems. However, it does not facilitate an examination 'into' the medical profession. The literature on the professions (for example, trait theory) examines the difference between professionals and other occupations or between professionals and their clients (e.g. Johnson, 1972) or the position of the medical profession within the division of labour (Freidson, 1986). However, the literature on the threat to the medical profession's dominance illustrates that the profession's powerful position has declined in the past 25 years but that these developments have been uneven within the profession. Although the literatures on the professions are important as they explain the dominance and the possible decline of the medical profession within an institution such as the English NHS, on their own they do not help us to further the aim of this study, which is to analyse how structural changes have influenced the intraprofessional relations between GPs and hospital consultants. So although this literature is important in informing any study of the medical profession, on its own its utility is limited when analysing the effects of structural change. A more effective framework to employ would be a structuralist approach such as that developed by Alford (1975) which I will discuss in detail.

HEALTH CARE POLITICS: USING ALFORD'S TYPOLOGY

Alford (1975) analysed various attempts to reform the health care system in New York City, arguing that the structured interests within the health service would mould new administrative devices to their own advantage. Health service reforms are usually precipitated by perceptions of a crisis, such crises usually being manufactured by interest groups either inside or outside the service. The purpose of this study is to analyse the impact on intraprofessional relations of a set of health policies, brought about by a so-called crisis in the NHS, which have altered the structure of the health system. For this purpose it is useful to use an approach such as Alford's idea of structural interests. This framework has been used by others in analysing a wide range of health policies in different countries including the conflicts of oriental medicine and pharmacy in Korea (Cho, 2000); the investigation of power and influence in health policy agenda-setting in Australia (Lewis and Considine, 1999); the effects of health care reforms on the health care systems of the United States and Britain (North, 1995); and most recently in studying the creation of primary care groups within the English NHS (North and Peckham, 2001).

In the late 1980s the then Conservative government responded to the perception of an NHS crisis with a set of radical health service reforms. Again, an administrative solution was used to correct what were seen by many as economic and political problems within the NHS, or as Hunter (1993) has argued:

> *The curiously never ending search for, and fascination with, technical solutions to what are at the end of the day political problems riven with value judgements that are not themselves susceptible to resolution through technical means or fixes.* (p. 8)

By using Alford's theoretical framework one is able to examine how the different interest groups within and around the health care system interact with and are affected by the health service reforms that have occurred during the 1990s in the English NHS. The role of the government in this milieu is a crucial one, as Alford (1975) states:

> *Government is not an independent power standing above and beyond the competing interest groups, but represents changing coalitions of elements drawn from various structural interests.* (p. 251)

These coalitions that Alford describes could also be made with certain groups within the structural interests, rather than with a whole structural interest, that is to say the government could team up with a particular section of a structural interest. When the NHS was created, Bevan, who then headed the Ministry of Health, teamed up with the hospital consultants and their royal colleges in order to overcome the objections to the creation of an NHS by GPs and their BMA representatives.

Alford identifies three such structural interests within a health care system, these being the dominant, challenging and repressed structural interests. He identified the medical profession as the professional monopolists, who represent the dominant structural interest served by the existing political, economic and social institutions (p. 14). Within the NHS context health service managers would be the corporate rationalizers, the challenging structural interests who attempt to introduce changes to the service that challenge the professional monopolists. Lastly, the repressed structural interests are represented in the USA by the section of the population who are either uninsured or without health care coverage (this structural interest does not transfer directly to the UK where the NHS provides universal coverage to its population). This structural interest requires political support in order to mount a challenge to the dominant structural interests within the health care system. These different groups will occupy different positions, adopt differing tactics and be affected in particular ways when changes are introduced.

Using Alford's political analysis of health services one can argue that the managerial reforms in the 1980s were an attempt by the government to strengthen the health service managers to enable them to challenge the dominant structural interests of the medical profession. This strategy by and large failed and the introduction of the 1991 reforms, which ushered in a more fundamental and radical approach to health service reform than had previously been attempted, can be viewed as a recognition of these earlier failings. Another thread of government health policy during the 1990s was the promotion of the idea of 'consumerism' into the NHS, which attempted to support the repressed structural interests of the public who were increasingly encouraged to question the medical profession and to act in a less deferential way to doctors. Initiatives such as the Patient's Charter, although fairly weak in practice, can be seen as policies by which the government attempted to lend support to the interests of the public within the health care system. The relative distribution of power among these groups will be influential in shaping the future performance of a health service; structural changes will also have an important impact on the distribution of power among the different structural interest groups (Hollingsworth, 1986). It should be stressed that Alford's typology is being put forward as an effective way in which to analyse government policy and not to suggest that the government consciously used such a framework when developing and implementing these policies.

Alford suggested that professional monopolizers derive their power through their interests being served by the social, political and economic structures in place (p. 14). This helps to explain why the medical profession is a conservative group, which will invariably attempt to resist change by neutralizing new structures or moulding new policies to their own advantage. The medical profession's power is not only evident in the conflicts where it has been triumphant but also in disputes that have never materialized. As Lukes (1974) argues: '*the most effective and insidious use of power is to prevent such conflict from arising in the first place*' (p. 23). That is to say that powerful groups do not always have to challenge changes since they can maintain the status quo by preventing reforms from even being contemplated or discussed.

Alford (1975) points out that the professional monopolizers are a heterogeneous group, within which battles periodically occur. However, he argues that the profession's fundamental common interests help them to unite so as to maintain their monopoly and safeguard their dominance within a heath system:

> *Their [professional monopolists] interests are thus affected differently by various programs of reform. But they share an interest in maintaining autonomy and control over the conditions of their work, and professional interests groups will – when that autonomy is challenged – act together in defense of that interest.* (p. 192)

What an elite theory such as Alford's often overlooks or oversimplifies are the different levels within an elite, and their differences in terms of power and influence (Harrison, Hunter and Pollitt, 1990). Although Alford allows for various different interest groups within each of the separate structural interests (p. 194), he perhaps underestimates the impact of these differences which common structural interests may not be able to keep in check. These divisions within the medical profession are particularly important in the British case. The interests of certain parts of the medical profession are served by different sections of society, or more importantly, are served by the more powerful sections of society. As Haywood and Alaszewski, writing in 1980, argued, this could be one of the reasons why the services for the old and the mentally ill have historically had fewer resources than acute medicine and general surgery, despite various government policies that have attempted to rectify this situation.

> *The problems [the DHSS attempting to prioritise elderly services] arise because the interests so affected will often be those of the most prestigious providers who will have considerable influence over local operational policies. There is a mismatch between the groups the DHSS would like to advantage, and the local distribution of power.* (p. 53)

There is always a dilemma for the professional monopolizers: on the one hand they must present a united front against outside threats and on the other they must allocate the rewards of such action among the profession. It is this dilemma which can lead to conflicts within the profession. Salter (1998) has argued that the divisions within the medical profession become more pronounced when it is on the offensive, suggesting that the profession's unified power is negative or blocking in nature. These internal conflicts become more pronounced in times of cost containment due to the fact that development in certain sectors can only occur through the reallocation of resources, a situation that creates winners and losers (Harrison and Pollitt, 1994). Although historically the medical profession has largely been able to contain and manage such internal conflicts, as in the case of the creation of the NHS during a time of expectant post-war prosperity, this may not be so in the future. Freidson (1994) has suggested that the cohesive forces that have held professions together may disappear altogether in the future as the profession's members cease to have a common outlook, arguing that the professions may undergo a process of internal combustion. It could be argued that the 1991 reforms, occurring at a time of both economic and ideological state retrenchment within the welfare field, followed by the 1999 NHS reforms, have managed to create a stratified medical profession, breaching its inner unity. This fits into a trend where '*Professionalism is being reborn in a hierarchical form in which every-day practitioners become subject to the control of professional elites*' (Freidson, 1994, p. 9).

Again, there is no suggestion that successive governments have had a predetermined plan which they have used to reform the service; instead, in common with other policy areas there has been a series of disjointed incremental changes which have been made in reaction to certain events. However, by analysing these policies in a coherent way one can examine the impact they have had on the NHS and on those within it, assessing in particular how the intraprofessional relations between hospital consultants and GPs have been changed by the 1991 and 1999 NHS reforms and what consequences for the NHS there could be in the future.

If one analyses the White Paper *Working for Patients* (Department of Health 1989g), there are various references made to the new role they envisaged for GPs under the fundholding scheme. The document points to the fact that GPs are perfectly placed within the health care system to improve services; that hospital consultants need to be ready to satisfy GPs' demands; and that GPs who enter the fundholding scheme will play an enhanced decision-making role within the NHS:

> *The relationships which GPs have with both patients and hospitals make them uniquely placed to improve patients' choice of good quality services . . . Hospitals and their consultants need a stronger incentive to look on GPs as people whose confidence they must gain if patients are to be referred to them . . . It [the GP fundholding scheme] will enable the practices which take part to play a more important role in the way in which NHS money is used to provide services for patients.* (Department of Health, 1989g, p. 48)

In Alford's terms it could be said that policy-makers viewed the GP fundholding scheme as a way of converting fundholding GPs into corporate rationalizers thus radically changing their relationship with hospital consultants and having possible implications for the development of the NHS. Alford's structural interests approach will be used to examine whether the 1991 NHS reforms converted GP fundholders into corporate rationalizers, challenging the hospital consultants who remained professional monopolists. Using Alford's (1975) words this study will assess whether GPs can be seen to

> *share an interest [with other corporate rationalizers] in maintaining and extending the control of their organization over the work of the professionals whose activities are key to the achievement of organizational goals [i.e. hospital consultants].* (p. 192)

Chapter 1 illustrated how the structures of the NHS throughout its history have tended to serve hospital medicine and hospital consultants, while GPs have made various attempts to challenge this dominance. The 1991 NHS reforms dramatically reformed the structural make-up of the service and it is important to examine how this has affected the relations between GPs and hospital consultants. To what extent did the restructured NHS allow GPs more successfully to challenge hospital consultants' dominance within the NHS? How did the 1999 NHS reforms further impact upon these new intraprofessional relations and what does the future policy environment hold for the medical profession?

It has been shown that there are various approaches to analysing power and power relations within the policy process. It has been argued that all the approaches have some explanatory value and that they all suffer from certain limitations. Alford's (1975) elite theory of structural interests has been presented as being an effective framework, which has been used by others, for analysing the intraprofessional powers of the medical profession. So as to further illustrate the applicability of Alford's structural interests framework in this study the following section will adopt it in order to analyse contemporary health policy in England.

THE NEW HEALTH CARE POLITICS?

One could interpret the health policies of the past 20 years as an example of successive governments following a predetermined plan for the NHS. However, this would be a mistake; instead, governments have taken a series of disjointed incremental decisions in response to events. Yet in order to understand the implications of these policies for the service, they need to be analysed in a coherent way. Following this approach it would be fruitful to analyse the various health policies directed towards the NHS since 1979 using Alford's (1975) political analysis of health services that has already been discussed above. In this context one can argue that the managerial reforms in the 1980s were an attempt by the state to create a cadre of health service managers who might control hospital doctors' organizational environment and thus challenge the dominant structural interests of the medical profession. These new managers can be recognized in Alford's description of corporate rationalizers:

> *The structural interest of corporate rationalization is represented by persons in top positions in "health" organizations . . . Their ideology stresses a rational, efficient, cost-conscious, co-ordinated health care delivery system.* (p. 204)

Although the introduction of management into the service may have had a cultural impact upon the medical profession, this strategy failed effectively to control hospital consultants and the profession continued its dominance within the NHS (Harrison, Hunter, Marnoch and Pollitt, 1992). Continuing with Alford's approach, the potentially fundamental reforms that the Conservative government embarked upon with the 1988 review of the NHS were legitimized by a perceived NHS crisis, a favoured tactic that is used by specific structural interests to make maximum political capital from a situation that had been present for some time. On the one hand the medical profession characterized the crisis as one of inadequate funding and thus sought more resources, and on the other hand the government characterized the origins of the crisis as structural and therefore embarked upon a structural reform of the service.

The introduction of the 1991 reforms can be viewed as recognition by the state of the earlier policy failings and their need to initiate a more fundamental and radical approach to health service reform that could build upon the NHS management structure that had been created in the 1980s. The 1991 package of NHS reforms introduced measures that were designed to assist hospital managers in their quest for greater control over the medical profession, particularly hospital consultants. As corporate rationalizers the hospital managers needed to be able to control their work places and thus control their employees, which is very difficult to do when they do not hold their most senior employees' contracts or have any mechanisms to monitor their employees' performance, which was the case for hospital consultants prior to the 1991 reforms. After 1991, hospital trust chief executives controlled hospital consultants' contracts and could to a limited extent require them to engage in medical audit, which potentially gave the corporate rationalizers further weapons to use in their efforts to manage the professional monopolists. These powers that were bestowed on hospital managers are echoed in Alford's (1975) discussion where he states that

> *They [corporate rationalizers] therefore attempt to convert professionals, mainly physicians, into employees and in a variety of ways to circumscribe their power in the hospital.* (p. 209)

However, the history of the Griffiths' reforms in the 1980s had shown hospital managers as being unable effectively to control hospital consultants no matter how much assistance the government gave them. This seemed still to be true in the 1990s as the medical profession was largely successful in neutralizing what could be considered the most threatening aspects of the 1991 reforms. Freidson's (1986) analysis of the nature of the medical profession's dominance, which was discussed earlier in this chapter, helps us to understand why this was the case.

As well as developing policies that would assist the health service managers in their role as corporate rationalizers, the 1991 reforms also created GP fundholders who were given the opportunity to develop managerial capabilities in the form of purchasers of health services. As fellow medics, the GP fundholders could represent the most effective managerial challenge to consultant clinicians (Mark and Scott, 1992). The research carried out for this study investigates to what extent the 1991 reforms empowered GPs to regulate the work of hospital consultants and thus to what extent they can be usefully viewed as the new agents of corporate rationalization within the NHS. Using Alford's language, this study will examine whether the internal contradictions among the professional monopolizers have led to a realignment of structural interests where GP fundholders have become the corporate rationalizers (p. 192–3).

During this same time, and later in the 1990s, the Conservative government promoted the idea of 'consumerism' within the health service and thereby attempted to support the repressed structural interests of the public who were encouraged to question the medical profession. Policies such as the Patient's Charter and the reviewed complaints' procedures (Department of Health, 1991; National Health Service Executive, 1995) were examples of this. Although much of the community's power has been illusory, it has at least compelled the medical profession to respond, if not to concede to their demands. The mere fact that such potentially radical reforms were being implemented at all is a clear sign of the medical profession's weakened position according to Lukes' (1974) analysis of power. Not only were such reforms being discussed but they were actually being implemented. Initiatives such as the Patient's Charter (Department of Health, 1991), although weak in practice, can be seen as a policy by which the state attempted to lend support to the interests of the public within the health care system. By 1997 it could be seen that many of the policies contained within the 1991 reforms had failed dramatically to allow health service managers or consumers to achieve a greater level of control over the medical profession. However, there were signs that GPs, particularly as part of fundholding practices, were having some impact upon the way hospital consultants carried out their work.

It has already been stated that the Labour government's 1999 health reforms were in many respects a continuation of those in 1991, particularly the most recent policy initiatives. Within PCTs GPs, along with other primary care professionals and managers, will no longer be restricted to commissioning just 20 per cent of their population's health service needs as was the case within the fundholding scheme; they will commission all the health services for their population. Within the new primary care organizations GPs will continue to have the potential to influence the way hospital consultants work and they will also be able to relocate certain hospital activities into primary care settings, particularly under the practice-based commissioning initiative (Department of Health, 2004a). It would seem from a policy analysis viewpoint that the 1999 reforms strengthen GPs' corporate rationalizer-type characteristics, although it can be argued that the reduced opportunities that the new primary care structures have for moving contracts among providers may act against this trend. Furthermore, the exhortations for commissioners and providers to co-operate may mean that GPs rejoin their hospital consultant colleagues as professional monopolizers. This potential may be strengthened by the fact that many of the Labour government's health policies are aimed at controlling the medical profession as a whole, rather than just one section of it. New organizations such as the Healthcare Commission and the National Institute for Clinical Excellence (NICE) together with initiatives such as National Service Frameworks (NSFs) and clinical governance can all be seen as ways of controlling how doctors carry out their work in both secondary and primary care. It remains to be seen whether the medical profession will attempt to present a united front in order to neutral-ize the potentially regulatory nature of these reforms and thus confirm Alford's view that the medical profession will ultimately act together to defend their common interests (pp. 192, 197).

In the context of Alford's structural interests framework it can be seen that the Labour government's health reforms could have vari-ous impacts on the three structural interests. On the one hand they build upon the Conservative government's policies that potentially cast GPs as the new corporate rationalizers within the NHS, and on the other they develop new initiatives that strengthen the hand of managers in their quest to control doctors within both secondary and primary care. Although the introduction of clinical governance has provided managers with a framework that they can potentially use to challenge the medical profession, many of the other 1999 initiatives do not directly give managers any substantial new powers. Instead, the Labour government has set up new agencies such as NICE and the Healthcare Commission in order to issue guidelines to health care professionals and monitor their performance respectively. These new national bodies contain managers, doctors and lay repre-sentatives in what can be seen as an attempt to create a new type of organization within the NHS. The next three chapters present empiri-cal findings that could act as a guide as to how the post-1999 reforms may influence the important intraprofessional relations of GPs and hospital consultants.

4

NEW PUBLIC MANAGEMENT ENTERS PRIMARY CARE

INTRODUCTION

The following three chapters will present the findings from two case studies into the intraprofessional relations of GPs and hospital consultants and further details of the methodology can be found in the appendix. These studies included two rounds of qualitative interviews and two surveys in the first case study of a general practitioner multifund and a further round of interviews in a second case study of a primary care group (PCG). The two case studies examined the impact of the 1991 NHS reforms developed by the Conservative administration and the emerging implications of the 1999 reforms enacted by the first Labour administration upon the intraprofessional relations of general practitioners and hospital consultants respectively. Upon analysis the data from the two case studies separated into three broad areas: first, the informants' perspectives of the fundholding scheme both during its actual operation and then after its abolition; second, the informants' perspectives upon the quality standards in particular and health care quality more generally; and last, the impact of the changing interface between primary and hospital care upon the intraprofessional relations of GPs and hospital consultants. These three areas will be discussed in Chapters 4, 5 and 6 respectively.

The nomenclature I have used for the data in these three chapters is fairly straightforward. The letters refer to the occupational group: GP is a general practitioner; C refers to a hospital consultant; and M denotes a manager. The numerals following the letter refer to the case study; Arabic numerals denote data from the first case study while the roman numerals refer to data from the second case study.

Before going on to examine the informants' perspectives of the fundholding scheme a brief background to the two case studies will be presented in order to provide the reader with a context.

THE CASE STUDIES

The first case study consisted of two rounds of face-to-face interviews, two questionnaire surveys and non-participant observations of contract setting meetings. The multifund under investigation came into being in 1994, making it part of the fourth wave of GP fundholders. There were 15 GP funds within the multifund; however, due to some grouping of surgeries, there was a total of 16 GP practices in all. There were 75 GPs involved with a total list size of 123,000 patients who made up about 20 per cent of the local district population, making it one of the larger multifunds according to an Audit Commission report (1996).

The multifund was financed from all the individual funds from which it was comprised. Each fundholding practice received a fundholding management allowance, 45 per cent of which went to the multifund's central management office, which was responsible for the majority of the management issues associated with fundholding such as contracting and invoicing. The individual fundholding practices were responsible for carrying out their individual data-entry tasks, but they had few of the wider management responsibilities allied to the fundholding scheme.

The 1991 NHS reforms allowed GP practices with list sizes above 3,000 to manage their own budgets and thus become GP fundholders. At the time of the first phase of data gathering (1995) there were three types of GP fundholding practices in operation: standard, community and total GP fundholding. The form of fundholding scheme in which the GP practice was located determined the cost and type of health services that the practice could purchase – this study investigated a group of standard fundholding practices. A GP practice that had a list size of over 5,000 could become a standard fundholder and would manage a budget (which was typically made up of a mix of capitation and historic expenditure). From this budget the practice paid for the drug costs, outpatient services and any day-case and inpatient services that cost below a total of £6,000. The local district health authority paid for other services such as accident and emergency and treatments costing over £6,000.

The first case study focused upon a standard GP fundholding

multifund. Typically multifunds consisted of various fundholding GP practices within a geographical area that grouped together to become a consortium or multifund; these groups could have different structures but they co-operated, to varying degrees, on the management issues associated with the fundholding scheme (Audit Commission, 1996).

The second case study obtained a snapshot of the perspectives of GPs, hospital consultants and health service managers of a new set of reforms that were being introduced by the new Labour government into the NHS. The PCG that was investigated in the second case study had 44 GPs who were located within 17 practices and the PCG had five staff working in its central office. Within the PCG, 12 of the practices were previously standard fundholders and one practice had been involved in a total purchasing pilot prior to the 1999 reforms. The PCG had an overall budget of £45 million and had a registered patient population of 90,000.

The limitations of this second case study must be recognized when considering these empirical chapters. This section of the overall research consisted of a small interview-based case study of one PCG and its main hospital trust provider. The interviews were carried out only a year after the PCG had been set up and hence the fundholding scheme for GPs had only recently been abolished. However, the perspectives on the fundholding scheme from these informants are particularly valuable as they had the benefit of a longer experience of this policy than those in the first case study.

An insight into the 'culture' of the multifund can be gained from examining some of the reasons given by the multifund GP informants for joining the fundholding scheme. The second case study sought to obtain a snapshot of the impact this policy had had upon the GP–hospital consultant relationship at a time when the scheme had been abolished. For these reasons informants from the second case study were asked about their experiences of the GP fundholding scheme and the internal market in general. They were able to look back on eight years' experience of the fundholding scheme, as opposed to the informants in the first case study who were commenting on a policy that was still developing. It is thus highly illustrative to group the perspectives from both case studies in one chapter so as to build up a picture of both the impact of the fundholding scheme during its existence and the early insights into the impact of its demise. In order to aid clarity the results from the first and second case study will be taken in turn.

THE FUNDHOLDING SCHEME AND THE
CONTRACTING PROCESS

The fundholding managers stated that the option of fundholding was preferred by the multifund GPs to locality commissioning because of the perceived freedoms offered to them by the fundholding scheme. It was stated that without actually having the money it was difficult to exercise control over purchasing; fundholding was seen as a way of controlling the money and therefore controlling purchasing. This was the way the multifund medical manager who was the GP leader of the multifund viewed the power of fundholding:

> *Rightly or wrongly if you're standing on a wallet, to put it crudely, you've got power. For 17 years we've been saying this is unsatisfactory, the minute you've got the money to contract for the service something gets done.* (GP8)

The fact of holding a budget was widely perceived among the fundholding GPs as being an effective leverage in negotiations of hospital services. Many of the fundholding GPs felt that this influence was absent before fundholding. The multifund GPs also felt that joining the fundholding scheme would extend this influence to their consultant colleagues, something that they felt had been lacking up to now, as this multifund GP explained:

> *. . . what I want to do is make sure our patients didn't have to wait ridiculously long times to be treated, that consultants were sensitive to the needs of our patients and would listen, which they never did before* (GP1).

A non-multifund fundholding GP, who had initially been sceptical of the fundholding scheme, also felt that it had given him greater influence over hospital services:

> *I wasn't particularly positive [about fundholding] but we are pleased with the results . . . we feel we've got more influence. I think it's meant that our voice is listened to more . . .* (GP4)

The GP informants felt that the alternative to fundholding would have been locality commissioning where GPs within a locality are involved in purchasing health services to varying degrees in conjunction with the local health authority (Wainwright, 1996) which, in their view, would not have given them the influence they enjoyed as fundholders. The following GP describes how it was their budget-holding capability that gave them the influence they now felt they had:

Well locality commissioning never took off really because ultim-
ately we [the GPs] had no say. Money mainly. That's the teeth. If
you can't have teeth, then forget it. You're simply creating another
tier of management, a lot of hot air, nothing gets done at the end
of the day. (GP1)

This evidence suggests that the perceived influence the multifund
GPs had was a function of the fundholding scheme rather than an
influence that derived from purely being in a multifund. Thus it was
the structural change within primary care and the fact that GPs could
control a budget that allowed them to exert demands upon hospital
services and challenge the working practices of hospital consultants.
Since fundholding was a voluntary scheme, joining it entailed an
active decision on the part of GPs who according to this evidence
joined because they were dissatisfied with the status quo. In Alford's
terms these GPs wanted to challenge the system thus becoming corporate rationalizers rather than preserve the status quo, which is the
desire of professional monopolizers (Alford, 1975, p. 195). At the
macro level the government in a process of corporate rationalization
created the conditions, via the introduction of the GP fundholding
scheme, for GPs to challenge the hospital consultants and at the micro
level GPs entered the new scheme, albeit somewhat reluctantly in this
case, in an attempt to exert more influence over hospital services.

However, the active nature of these GPs' decisions to enter the
fundholding scheme needs to be questioned as GPs in the multifund
described themselves as 'reluctant fundholders'. They were fourth-
wave fundholders rather than joining the fundholding scheme on
earlier waves. A multifund manager had no illusions about the
majority of the GPs' lack of interest in the management element of
the fundholding scheme. This is how she perceived the majority of
the GPs within the multifund:

We've bashed our heads against a brick wall to a degree about
trying to get non-interested GPs interested in the process of fund-
holding. They're not and the thing that we have to keep reminding
ourselves as well is that they went into fundholding in the fourth
wave, they were not born again fundholders, they were not inter-
ested most of them at the beginning. They went in very reluctantly
because they didn't want to be in the wrong tier of society as far as
their patients were concerned and having done that that's why they
went into it in a multifund and there are still lots of them who say
if the multifund didn't exist I would have no way considered
fundholding on my own. (M7)

This view was supported by an Audit Commission report (1996) on fundholding which stated that multifund-type structures had encouraged some GPs to join the fundholding scheme who would otherwise have been reluctant to do so owing to the management responsibilities involved in the scheme. This particular multifund was made up of GPs who in the main were individually hesitant to take on the many management responsibilities that they saw as being associated with the fundholding scheme. The following multifund GP articulated a widespread view among the multifund GPs:

> *None of us would have undertaken fundholding individually without some help, outside help because most of it is management and we didn't feel we were management trained.* (GP6)

The administrative burden that he perceived to be connected to the fundholding scheme was given as the main reason for not entering the scheme by the non-fundholding GP informant:

> *The one very important reason was that we felt threatened by the extra administrative workload it would involve . . . None of the three partners felt that they wanted to take on the additional administrative workload.* (GP2)

This view would tend to confirm that the perceived management workload associated with the fundholding scheme acted as a deterrent to membership for some GPs. The multifund approach was seen as one way of overcoming this management hurdle.

The main reason cited by the multifund GP informants for finally entering the fundholding scheme was their fear that their patients may lose out as a consequence of being outside the scheme. This multifund GP expressed a common argument for joining the fundholding scheme as part of a multifund:

> *Overall we weren't in favour [of becoming fundholders] and then we saw everybody else going in and we expected that our patients could become disadvantaged if we didn't join. And so we went reluctantly into fundholding and because we didn't really want to be too involved in the bureaucracy of it, the multifund suggestion came up . . .* (GP7)

As well as a perceived inevitability of fundholding the multifund GP informants also felt that joining the scheme would enable them to improve the hospital services that they felt to be under-performing. The following GP view was widespread among the multifund GPs:

We decided to go fundholding because we felt that it was an inevitable move within general practice in this area and we were unhappy with certain services available for our patients . . . (GP3)

The GPs within this multifund had a good working relationship with the local hospital doctors and another of the reasons given for forming a multifund was to support their local hospital. However, it was recognized by the GP informants that the desire to support the local provider blunted the internal market's competitive thrust, which purchasers such as GP fundholders might wish to use in attempts to make providers improve or adapt their services. This point was expressed by one multifund GP:

. . . it's always been the ethos behind it [the multifund] that we actually want to support our hospitals, then they know when we come up requesting various quality controls our hands are somewhat tied anyhow because we want to see a thriving local hospital. (GP6)

The comment indicates that competition outside the metropolitan areas of England was limited because purchasers in these situations, like this multifund, were keen to support their local providers due to the lack of alternatives. The multifund did exert some pressure on its providers, as will be illustrated later in this chapter, but competition was far from fierce in this area of the country.

Entering the fundholding scheme entailed participating in the contracting process. The quality standards were explored in the first case study within the broader context of the contracting process. Most of the informants were ambivalent about the importance and relevance of a contracting process for the delivery of health care, regarding it as an unnecessary and rather abstract paper chase. A health authority manager reflected this view, stating that contracts were often

. . . interesting bits of paper to refer to but no one ever does, and doesn't necessarily bear any relation to what is happening on the ground. (M2)

The consultant informants who were in general unaware of what was contained within the contracts echoed this view. The following consultant articulated a widespread view among the consultant informants:

I think quite a lot of the consultants in any hospital, not just this one are unaware of the niceties of the contracting process . . .

*some people are probably totally unaware of what quality stand-
ards have been negotiated or of what target numbers have been
negotiated.* (C5)

A multifund manager stated that contracting had meant:

A lot of paperwork, a lot of chasing around . . . (M7)

However, the GPs expressed a more ambivalent view towards contracting: on the one hand they could see certain disadvantages associated with the process such as the added administration that some
informants pointed out, while on the other they felt it gave them the
leverage over the provider unit which, in their view, they did not have
prior to contracting. One multifund GP gave an example of the
perceived leverage the contracting process gave them:

*. . . what happened was that our intention to purchase outpatient
services from one other hospital led to a major review of the way
that the department worked . . .* (GP1)

A senior hospital consultant who was able to give a concrete example
of how a service had been forced to improve due to the contracting
process confirmed this perception:

*Some specialties, notably ophthalmology, have reduced the time
for patients to be seen as an outpatient and reduced the time for
patients to come in for day case cataracts dramatically over the
last 18 months because there's been pressure, pressure through the
contracts.* (C5)

Another consultant who was the clinical director of surgery cor-
roborated this view. He stated that

*. . . if you look at eyes and ENT there's been an enormous improve-
ment in performance in the last year, 18 months, those sort of
issues are very much better. There's a large increase in throughput,
the waiting list is coming down, 30% reduction, they are important
quality measures and I think the contracting process has got a lot
to take credit for over that.* (C6)

Interestingly a hospital consultant felt that the contracting process
could also bring them certain benefits. This consultant thought that
if a particular service was valued by GPs they could use this fact to
gain more resources from the trust management:

*So I think in many ways if there's something that the general
practitioners, patients need/want then your chances of getting it
are better in the contracting process.* (C1)

These data suggest that although some managers and clinicians saw contracting as a time-consuming administrative burden, it was also recognized that the process could be a vehicle for effecting change. GPs saw the contracting process as enabling them to exert change in hospital services and hospital consultants also felt that they could use the contracting mechanism to highlight deficiencies that needed to be addressed. This evidence can be viewed in one of two ways: either as an example of both branches of the medical profession using and moulding new structures to their own advantage as suggested by Alford (1975) – both GPs and hospital consultants exhibiting professional monopolist type characteristics – or as the result of the professional monopolists, in this case the hospital consultants, allying themselves with the new corporate rationalizers, the fundholding GPs, in order to gain more resources and legitimacy (Alford 1975, p. 209). The concluding chapter will consider these issues more fully in the light of all the empirical evidence that is presented.

A health authority manager explained why he felt the contracting process had enabled the GP fundholders to achieve these changes. He argued that GP fundholders had achieved a greater flexibility in the contracting process than health authorities because they purchased on the margins, a point that was made by a health authority manager in the second case study. He also attributed the GPs' success in improving services to the fact that they were more closely connected to the hospital consultants, stating:

> *I think certainly nationally they have been seen to be more nimble footed in purchasing and contracting than health authorities. Partly because they have been able to operate more at the margins but also because significantly they have a more direct clinical link with, particularly the consultants in the hospitals.* (M1)

COMMENT

These examples illustrate that the GPs in this multifund were reluctant to join a fundholding scheme whose associated management responsibilities were regarded by them as threatening and time-consuming. On the other hand they saw the multifund structure as a way to gain the perceived advantages of fundholding without what they saw as the management burdens of the scheme. The multifund GPs felt that joining the fundholding scheme would allow them to support their local hospital trust and also improve certain services. Although many informants saw the contracting process as an extra layer of bureaucracy, the process was also seen as a mechanism by which GPs could influence hospital services. The data illustrate that both GPs and consultants credited the contracting process with allowing them to make improvements in certain hospital services, although it should also be noted that certain GPs, particularly those who remained outside the fundholding scheme, felt uneasy about what they saw as the commercial nature of the contracting process.

THE END OF THE FUNDHOLDING SCHEME

One of the aims of the second case study was to examine how permanent any of the changes that resulted from the 1991 reforms would be once the fundholding practices were absorbed into PCGs as part of the post-1997 Labour reforms. It was therefore important to seek these informants' experiences of the GP fundholding scheme and the internal market. These perceptions would be particularly insightful, as the informants would be commenting upon a policy from beginning to end.

All the informants in the second case study stated that the introduction of fundholding had resulted in GPs' views having a greater impact upon hospital clinicians and managers. Hospital consultants and managers from this trust had set up a marketing operation that actively canvassed the opinions of local GPs. The following consultant who was involved in this marketing strategy described the initial lack of communication between the commissioners and providers of services that had occurred when the internal market had first been introduced:

> *Not in any, how shall I say, coherent way. No, there was no established or formalised system for us getting out to display our services, and at the same time get feedback from our local purchasers as to what we wanted.* (Ci)

This consultant then went on to describe how the trust reacted to the loss of income from local GP fundholders who had moved certain contracts to alternative providers. It is worth quoting him at length on the approach the trust adopted and why the trust arranged a reception for the local GPs as it demonstrates the importance that was placed upon GP fundholders by hospital trusts and hence the influence the GP fundholders could exert on these hospitals and their consultants:

> ... *when we'd lost a lot of fundholding income and we decided to set up a proper marketing strategy ... we got our act together, and a lot of the traditional long wait specialties like ENT, ortho-paedics, urology, got their act together with some, you know, good partnerships between the clinicians and the management to really improve accessibility. And my role with the marketing team was to set up various forums to meet the GPs and make sure that they knew we were actively listening and were taking on board what they were saying, and within a year we'd got all that fundholding income back ... the first major event we held was a highly suc-cessful forum at one of the local hotels where we just had all the key consultants in, all the lead clinicians who were running ser-vices, and a lot of clinical directors, and any interested consultant was there. I mean we had them literally all round the place with their stands with all the leaflet information for how to access the service and, you know, what service would be provided. Managers there as well, but the consultants were there on view, we had masses of GPs come in. It was held one evening, obviously there was food and drink, and the feedback from that was phenomenal, because the GPs thought it was brilliant that they, in one evening, could go along and chat to any consultant that they wanted to.* (Ci)

Thus the loss of income from GP fundholders forced the trust to address the GPs' concerns by actively listening to them, which in turn forced the hospital consultants to engage with the local GP fundholders. A fundholding GP informant described his reactions to these initiatives:

> *And there'd be meals and there'd be sort of smoked salmon recep-tions and all sorts of bleeding things. And, you know, meet the consultant, sell the service, sell the service, sell the service ... And this happened for the first time. And we thought, 'Well, you know, we've never had meetings before.'* (GPi)

These informants' accounts illustrate that the approach taken by the trust was certainly new and one that would not have occurred had it not been for the introduction of the internal market and GP fund-holders' ability to contract for certain hospital services. These data demonstrate how structural change forced hospital consultants to listen more closely to their GP colleagues than they had in the past, giving GPs the opportunity to influence the way hospital consultants provided services.

A trust manager also recognized the importance of such meetings between GPs and consultants:

> *But if you can get them [consultants and GPs] in the same room and usually provide sandwiches and a parking space, two key things, then you can often get solutions.* (Mi)

The above account recognizes the key position the medical profession as a whole holds within the health care service.

Although GPs and hospital consultants communicated with each other before the 1991 reforms, their exchanges tended to relate to clinical issues rather than to how services were organized. A senior consultant described how he thought the nature of communications between GPs and consultants had changed since the advent of the internal market and the GP fundholding scheme:

> *I think before the 1991 reforms, there was very little [communication], I mean there was clinical communication. There wasn't much communication around how the Health Service was run.* (Cii)

The nature of communication between GPs and hospital consultants had been perceived to change as a consequence of the 1991 reforms from what had been a purely clinical discussion to one that also included the organization of the health care system. This marks an important change as it means that GPs were entering discussions about hospital organization that had previously been solely the domain of hospital consultants.

A GP who was a member of the PCG board also thought that prior to the fundholding scheme there had been little communication between GPs and consultants and that it was the introduction of the scheme that had spawned such initiatives. In particular he felt that it was the fact that GP fundholders had financial powers that made consultants listen to them, thus echoing the views of the fundholding GPs from the first case study:

> *GP fundholding acted as a catalyst to bring the two sides together. Before GPs and consultants didn't talk to each other professionally . . . The consultants wouldn't have come to the table without GPs having the budget. Because a reasonable amount of resources were with the GPs it forced the consultants to consult with the GPs. 75% of GPs were fundholders [in this area] so they had to be*

consulted. They had to come to the table . . . Only lip service was
paid to them without a budget. (GPii)

In common with the consultants in the first case study, these hospital consultants also felt that the fact that GP fundholders held a
budget meant that they could exert real influence upon hospital services. The following consultant explains how the fact that GPs
became budget holders focused the minds of hospital clinicians:

> *. . . you got the fundholders actually with the money in their hands*
> *to say, 'Well we've got this budget to have our patients have their*
> *hips operated on and we're gonna shop around so we can find*
> *somewhere which will give us a decent service, you know, will do*
> *the job but also do it as quickly as possible, because our patients*
> *are suffering.' And I mean I think that concept focused a lot*
> *of minds really . . . I think GPs voting with their feet and their*
> *wallets, if you like, well the practices' wallets of course, that*
> *focused minds a bit.* (Ci)

The other consultant informants echoed this consultant's account
and they illustrate how GP fundholders' budget-holding quality
enabled them to challenge some of the working practices of their
hospital consultant colleagues. This situation of GP fundholders
finds resonance with Alford's description of corporate rationalizers
who attempt to restrict the power and control the work of hospital
doctors (Alford, 1975, p.209).

The consultants that were interviewed felt that they personally
would ultimately be affected if GP fundholders did move their contracts to other providers. This is how the same consultant described
his perceived vulnerability to fundholding GPs:

> *I think ultimately what was happening was everything was becom-*
> *ing very transparent so you'd got, as I say, GPs being very vocal,*
> *saying, 'This is just not good enough, and we can get it done much*
> *quicker down the road.' And you'd got the Trust management*
> *saying, 'Christ, those guys are going down the road. We're losing*
> *all this money and you guys in whatever, I mean if this carries*
> *on, if our contract's going to be downsized then the number of*
> *consultants is going to be downsized.'* (Ci)

Although this consultant's views were not an isolated one, the
limited nature of this second case study should be recognized. However, the consultant accounts vividly illustrate how fundholding GPs
were effectively challenging the work of hospital consultants.

During the life of the GP fundholding scheme commentators had noted differences in the treatment received by patients from fund-holding and non-fundholding GPs (Dixon, 1994; Dixon *et al.*, 1994; Dowling, 1997). The multifund GP informants also pointed to the detrimental impact upon their patients of staying outside the GP fundholding scheme as a reason for entering the scheme. These perceptions were confirmed by a non-fundholding GP informant who felt there were differences between how he and his patients were treated during the fundholding period – he felt that there had been inequities between fundholding and non-fundholding GPs:

> . . . *when I talked to colleagues and attending other meetings, they are talking about their patients being seen earlier. And they have more relationship with the consultant than the non-fundholders.* (GPiii)

It was not only the non-fundholding GP informant who perceived a two-tier system within general practice for the duration of the fund-holding scheme; fundholding GPs also recognized that the scheme had created this, as this GP stated:

> . . . *and there were unethical plus sides [to being a fundholding GP]. Yeah, our patients got treated really quickly and they were pleased as punch. So, you know, that's a plus side . . . Well as long as you were a fundholder, then you were given automatic priority over non-fundholders. And it was as simple as that.* (GPi)

A consultant informant also stated that he had sensed a tension between the fundholding and non-fundholding GPs, which he felt was rooted in the perceived inequity of the fundholding system:

> . . . *the feeling was amongst the hospital clinicians that GPs who were fundholders out there, were a little bit more demanding than non-fundholders, and this actually, in our opinion, certainly in my personal opinion, created a rift, and unhappiness between the GPs out there and between the fundholders and the non-fundholders. I felt that when I went out there talking to GPs, which were both fundholders and non-fundholders, I could see that there are tensions there.* (Ciii)

However, this same consultant went on to stress the fact that the relations between consultants and GPs were good regardless of the GPs' fundholding status:

> *I have a fantastic relationship with all my GPs here, and that's*

irrespective of the fact that they're fundholders or non-fundholders.
(Ciii)

Although all the GP informants recognized that the fundholding scheme had produced inequalities between patients registered with fundholders and those on the list of non-fundholding GPs, they also all felt that the scheme had enabled the fundholding GPs to improve the services they could offer to their patients. One fundholding GP explained what he had been able to achieve for his patients under the fundholding scheme:

> . . . *when we were fundholding, we could get things done for our patients. We could be innovative when it came to our patients, so we organised phlebotomy services, counselling, physiotherapy, dietetics, speech therapy, and we negotiated very good deals. And the savings we were able to use by negotiating additional deals. And we didn't have waiting lists for modern and complex treatments. My partners and I would have preferred to have kept going with fundholding. But, of course, it wasn't fair, wasn't equitable, and it was too costly.* (GPiv)

This GP's account illustrates the tension that was present within the fundholding scheme; the scheme produced tangible benefits for their patients, but these benefits were achieved at the cost of other patients who were registered with non-fundholding GP practices.

The first case study found that in the early days of GP fundholding the providers' perceptions were that fundholding GPs were being unrealistic in their demands of secondary care. However, a hospital consultant who also expressed this view in this phase recognized that that these types of GPs were in the minority:

> *I think certainly one or two practices really felt they had the upper hand and tried to push everything. Other practices were very realistic and there was a meeting of minds and they realised our problems and we realised their problems.* (Civ)

As has already been stated, the consultants also felt that GP fundholders had helped to focus the minds of the hospital consultants and managers on the service they were providing in secondary care. The threat that GP fundholders had of moving their contracts to another trust meant that the consultants had to adapt their services to respond to local GPs' demands. These perceived threats not only resulted in the marketing exercises that have been already described, the consultants also felt that due to these demands the quality of the service they offered had improved. The following two hospital consultants gave concrete examples of these improvements:

> . . . *it may be heresy, but actually it [the fundholding scheme] was very good for us. Because we did a lot of outreach clinics and quite a lot of initiatives for them [fundholding GPs], our actual waiting times for out-patient appointments and our in-patient waiting list times improved considerably.* (Civ)

> . . . *the fundholders have been able to refer to whoever they want to refer and purchase services from a distant hospital. So I mean that's raised the level of our quality of care, certainly in terms of how responsive it is and how well it matches up to a neighbouring Trust. So I mean the whole internal market achieved that.* (Cv)

This evidence suggests that fundholding GPs were able successfully to challenge the working practices of hospital consultants and make the hospital service more responsive to the needs of GPs and their patients, again displaying corporate rationalizer-type characteristics.

The managers interviewed from both the health authority and the PCG also recognized that GP fundholders had managed to make positive changes to the health service. However, they pointed out that this might have been because they were not responsible for commissioning all the services and this allowed them to be more flexible than health authorities that were responsible for commissioning the whole range of health services for their population. Other commentators have argued that GP fundholders were delegated the easy 20 per cent of purchasing while the health authorities were responsible for purchasing the far more difficult 80 per cent of health services (Light, 1998). The manager informants felt that things might be different when GPs in primary care trusts had to commission all the health services for their population. When asked if giving the GPs a budget had turned hospital services round, a health authority manager stated that

> *Yes, it did. But it worked on the margins, and that's why it was possible to turn it around. What we're talking about a lot of the time is not working on the margins but working on the absolute mainstream. So if you look at where fundholding applied, the range of procedures for fundholding were pretty small actually.* (Mi)

The PCG manager made observations similar to those of the health authority manager:

I think GP fundholding didn't expose GPs to the realities of commissioning. They were protected. They only had a range of services that they commissioned . . . So I think that they had a cushy life as fundholders. They need to be exposed to the reality of the overall commissioning system. (Miii)

The points made by these two managers are of vital importance since primary care trusts (PCTs) will not be commissioning selected services for their patients, they will be responsible for commissioning and providing the whole range of health services. Although the experiences of the GP fundholding scheme give an insight to how PCGs and PCTs might perform, the crucial differences between the two models, as described by these two managers, must be recognized.

The GPs, hospital consultants and the managers interviewed all agreed that the fundholding scheme had raised the profile of GPs, particularly in relation to their hospital consultant colleagues. A senior hospital consultant explained how in the past there had been a perceived difference in status between the two branches of medicine:

. . . there was always a feeling of a difference between hospital doctors and primary care doctors really . . . on the one hand, hospital consultants thought they were slightly more special than GPs. And there might have been a bit of inverted reaction to that on the part of GPs. (Cii)

One ex-GP fundholder explained how he felt this situation had been changed by the introduction of the GP fundholding scheme and was being continued with the creation of PCGs:

But I think certainly the fundholding model and the PCG model have all meant that GPs should have better self esteem when it comes to the way they are perceived in relation to consultants. (GPiv)

All the hospital consultants that were interviewed felt that the introduction of fundholding had raised the GPs' status in relation to them. One consultant said:

I think when the fundholding came up . . . and there's no doubt that a lot of GPs enjoyed their new found power, and probably after years of being felt they were being looked down upon by hospitals and consultants in particular, you know, they felt it was time to sort of redress the balance, and I can fully understand that and don't blame them for it. (Ci)

All the consultants that were interviewed felt that the days of the all-powerful hospital consultant had disappeared in the past ten years. This was how one consultant expressed this widely held view:

I think it has changed tremendously . . . the GPs perhaps ten years ago did not have much say, and the consultants were felt to be, and I must say, wrongly at times, felt to be all mighty and powerful, do anything and get away with anything . . . But generally speaking, I think there has been a shift where we now feel, as a consultant body, that GPs have more say on how the patients are provided with the care that they need, rather than the consultants. (Ciii)

The above data point to a subtle change in emphasis where GPs have a greater control over the type of services that their patients receive and the way that these services are provided. Out-reach clinics are a good example of this and are an area that will be considered at the end of this chapter.

The consultants interviewed no longer saw GPs as failed doctors; they were now seen as specialists in their own right. This is how the same consultant informant described what he saw as the new GP:

I think, again historically, it may well be true that people who went out into general practice were the ones who could not progress well in hospital practice. That may be a historical fact. I'm not so sure as to whether it is still true . . . Now I think this new breed of GP and this new breed of consultant, we're not going to have people out there in primary care who couldn't make it. (Ciii)

Another hospital consultant very much echoed these views:

. . . the quality of the people going into primary care seems to have improved enormously. And as I say, their career structure is now matching that of any medical specialty. (Civ)

The health service managers also felt that the fundholding scheme had changed the power balance between GPs and hospital consultants in favour of the GPs. A trust manager felt that the ability to influence consultant behaviour was a major reason why GPs had taken part in the fundholding scheme. He felt that

Fundholders salivated when they got fundholding status. The two things they wanted were to try and influence consultant behaviour, because the consultants always thought they were up here and the GPs down there. (Mi)

Although the health authority manager was less convinced by the actual impact GP fundholders could have on hospital consultants, she did concede that some changes had occurred due to the introduction of the GP fundholding scheme:

> *. . . whilst I don't think that they could control in any way the clinicians, secondary care clinicians, because I mean there is still a lot of tensions around power with those clinicians, certainly they can change the nature of the debate and their level of influence will consequently be rather different . . . so it did start changing that and the consultants were having to come along and talk to the fundholding board and say, you know, 'We really would like to do this.' So it started changing it then. But I mean that status issue, I would say, still remains to some extent I think, though they're better at talking about things.* (Mii)

The evidence from this manager is important as it suggests that although structural change within primary care has allowed GPs to enter the debate with hospital consultants the balance of power has perhaps not shifted towards the GPs as far as some of the other informants may have indicated.

A PCG manager felt that consultants had had to change their mode of engagement with GPs when they had become fundholders. This manager stated:

> *I think that consultants do see that the GPs are increasingly important in the whole scheme of things, and do have to engage with them more closely and more correctly. And so I think they are seeing that they have to change to work with the GPs.* (Miii)

The data from these interviews illustrate that all the informants recognized that the fundholding scheme had increased GPs' power; however, we must be cautious to not overstate the extent of this upon GPs' influence. Moreover, the data from these interviews also illustrate that there was a feeling among both GPs and consultants themselves that the standing of hospital consultants within hospitals had changed in the past ten years. This is to say that not only had they lost status vis-à-vis GPs but they had also decreased in importance in relation to a hospital consultant 25 years ago. This is how one GP informant described his changing perception of hospital consultants:

> *They're not as entrepreneurial and eminent as they were. They're actually perceived as workers, important workers, but they actually have a contractual relationship with the Trust, and there's an expectation they will satisfy their contract.* (GPiv)

A hospital consultant agreed with the GP's perception, stating simply that

> *We're an employee same as anybody else.* (Civ)

These last two comments are important as they indicate that the medical profession as a whole has lost influence and this has allowed a certain amount of re-stratification to occur *within* the profession.

COMMENT

It can be seen that the informants in the second case study echoed many of the views expressed about the GP fundholding scheme by the informants in the first case study. There are also certain important differences. These informants did not speak as much of confrontation between primary and secondary care as those in the first case study. This may be to do with a different environment or, more likely, that as the GP fundholders matured in their role as purchasers they became more realistic about what secondary care could do. Equally, the hospital consultants recognized that there were changes that they could and did make that had improved the quality of the service they provided. Another important difference in the data from this case study was that all the GPs recognized the inequalities in service provision that the GP fundholding scheme had created, which was not as evident from the informants in the first case study.

One of the activities that mushroomed under the GP fundholding scheme was the provision of outreach clinics. This was an area that did not form part of the interview schedule but was a theme that was raised in the interviews by the informants as an example of one of the effects of the GP fundholding scheme and it was an area that was thus pursued. This theme proved to be an important example by which to investigate the intraprofessional relations of GPs and hospital consultants and it is therefore instructive to examine the informants' perspectives of this development in both case studies.

OUTREACH CLINICS

The growing number of outreach clinics is a good example of how the various professionals held contrasting views of certain health service developments. These clinics were frequently mentioned by GPs in the first case study as characterizing a good quality service for patients and something that the fundholding scheme had enabled them to promote. The following comment by a multifund GP illustrates this widespread view:

> *Well we had probably the one advantage that I can see of fundholding in that we brought more outreach clinics so the hospital now has more consultant clinics ... I mean certainly it's an improvement that patients can get more seen more local. That is a distinct improvement. These outreach clinics whether they're good from an organisation point of view. They're very good for patients. Patients like them rather than travelling all the way up to [their local hospital].* (GP7)

The development of outreach clinics was often seen as one of the biggest advantages of the fundholding scheme. The following multifund GP used outreach clinics as an example of what can be done as a fundholder and bemoans that little else had changed in her view:

> *Well in certain areas we've been able to make improvements because we've introduced in-house clinics. So the ability to do that has actually enabled us to direct services ourselves so that we get who we want doing the clinics, when we want and a much shorter waiting time for the patients and in many cases I think they get a better service ... So that's good but on the other hand the same principle has not enabled us to do all that we had wanted to do. It has not enabled us to do anything about all of the problem areas so we've still got patients waiting months and months and months for certain specialties which we don't seem to be able to influence and which I think we had thought we would be able to influence especially as a consortium ... Those specialties that were good and we were totally happy with are still good and probably even better. But those ones where you would have liked to have done something, you still haven't done anything.* (GP3)

However, not all the GPs felt that the growth of outreach clinics was a beneficial development within primary care. One multifund GP had reservations about these clinics; she felt they were restrictive and doubted their cost-effectiveness:

> *I have great reservations because I feel that, first of all it limits who you refer people to. Actually if you had a surgeon coming down to do a clinic between 6.00 and 7.00 once a week you are actually going to be limited to referring all your surgical cases to*

him and there is specialisation within the surgery so I think that's better really . . . And I also feel that at the end of the day you're actually paying someone twice for doing the same job, which I think morally, I'm very against. (GP6)

The hospital consultant informants shared this GP's views. The consultants who were interviewed were dubious about the benefits of these clinics; they felt that on the whole it was generally an inappropriate service to offer when there was so much sub-specialization in modern medicine. The following consultant also stated what he thought the incentives for such services might be, very much echoing the views of the dissenting GP informant:

Now we're getting into the realms of sub-specialisation in general surgery in a very big and very rapid manner and the GPs have got to understand this process and that is one of the reasons where individual consultants popping off to do outreach clinics is in my judgement beginning to be counter-productive. It's a convenience for the GPs because it's cheap. It's a convenience for the patients because it's local. It's a bonus for the consultants because they get backhanders but actually whether that's the right way of doing it I really don't know . . . You come and do an outreach clinic in my surgery which gives me good kudos with my patients and you can have all my private practice. (C6)

This same hospital consultant gave a concrete example of what he saw as the disadvantages of such arrangements:

I saw a lady who'd been waiting for a month to see me with a breast lump because that was the next time I was going to be there whereas we'd have seen her within 2 days at the hospital if she'd come up to the referral practice. So there is a down side. (C6)

It was recognized by most of the informants who mentioned the issue of outreach clinics that there were two sides to the issue which are important to appreciate. The multifund manager stated the advantages, as she saw them, of these clinics:

It depends on your point of view but some would argue that they should be in the hospital, others will argue that it's perfectly reasonable. They see so many more patients because they're in a different set-up. The patients are pleased to be there in a GP's surgery where they feel their doctor has given them the appointment to be seen at their own doctor's. People don't DNA [Did Not Attend] or if they can't make an appointment they ring and say so that's given to somebody else, so you get very little wastage. And it's cheaper, because you've not got all the hospital overheads and things. (M7)

However, the medical manager of the multifund felt that outreach clinics were a good development but only when they were properly set up and had the necessary funding:

For instance you need £50,000 worth of equipment to set up a proper ophthalmology or ENT outreach clinic as opposed to just having a consultant come along and go into a general practice surgery with nothing more than a case and a white coat, which, in my view, is not the correct way of doing outreach clinics although it is done. (GP8)

Virtually all the consultant informants in the second case study raised the issue of outreach clinics, although it did not feature in many of the GP accounts. One consultant felt that it was a good development, although he regretted the uni-practice focus that characterized it under the fundholding scheme:

. . . we in fact audited one of my [outreach] clinics and presented it to our health authority. The numbers were small, but what it showed, the patient satisfaction was much greater, the waiting time was non-existent, the waiting time was as long or as frequent as clinics were. . . . We'd drawn up guidelines, protocols, what to refer, what not to refer, and over a cup of tea whenever we got together, there was a lot of problems solved, which would have otherwise come into the clinic. I think the main disadvantage was it was not available to the whole population. (Ciii)

Another senior consultant agreed with this disadvantage:

I think the outreach under fundholding was perhaps not the right way because it was very much practice-focused instead of, you know, locality or population focused. (Cii)

The inequities of outreach clinics were also raised by one of the PCG GP informants who had not entered the fundholding scheme. When asked if his practice had had access to outreach clinics he responded that:

We didn't have one . . . because we were not fundholding. (GPiii)

However, as a GP he perceived many of the advantages that were mentioned by the multifund GP to the development of outreach clinics:

> *. . . the reasons for outreach clinics is that they meet with the patient and the patients are seen in the local environment where they like to be seen in the general practice rather than being in hospital. And they have been seen quicker. So when the consultant comes and see a patient in general practice, at least the inappropriate or unwarranted referrals could be minimised with it. So that at least the outpatients' clinic can be done within the practice. It saves a lot of resources especially financially. Patients who go to hospital cost more than seeing them in general practice.* (GPiii)

Another consultant felt that the outreach clinics had become of limited value since the teaching component of the clinics soon disappeared. This view is more in line with the research that has been carried out on the value of outreach clinics in primary care (Bailey, Black and Wilkin, 1994). This is how one consultant viewed his experience of providing outreach clinics:

> *. . . the GPs always asked for outreach clinics on sort of two main bases. One was that it was the locality and close for the patient, and the second was it was teaching for them. Well the teaching for them dropped off very rapidly, they never ever attended . . . And I think in the end we began to feel that really it wasn't a good use of manpower.* (Civ)

The data concerning the issue of outreach clinics illustrate that what constitutes a good-quality health service is dependent upon where the clinician is situated within the service (Baeza and Calnan, 1999). GPs who are unsure about a patient's condition value a short waiting time for an outpatient's appointment while the consultants feel that the final outcome is the important quality indicator. These points were reflected in the data that suggest that in general GPs viewed the development of consultants coming to their surgeries to run clinics far more positively than hospital consultants. The growth in the number of outreach clinics was an example of how GPs managed to influence the work of hospital consultants under the fundholding scheme. However, the evidence on outreach clinics from the second case study illustrates that these were of limited use due to their uni-practice focus, which constituted an inequity of access for patients who were not registered with fundholding practices.

SUMMARY

The fundholding GPs in the first case study were initially reluctant to join the fundholding scheme. The factors that encouraged them to enter the scheme were a fear that their patients may lose out if they remained outside fundholding and a desire to influence hospital services and hospital consultants. The mechanism that would give them this influence in their view was their budget-holding capacity that they could use via the contracting process. When they did enter the scheme they went in as part of a multifund in order to avoid the managerial aspects of fundholding. The lack of interest on the part of most multifund GPs in the managerial aspects of fundholding, which can be viewed as the tools of corporate rationalization, had an impact on their level of involvement in the mechanics of the scheme and is perhaps an indication of their general reluctance to use the instruments of corporate rationalization. This reluctance on the part of most of the GPs may have been one of the reasons why the potential levers of influence were not used effectively. As far as the hospital consultants were concerned they were also disengaged from the mechanics of contracting and were largely unaware of the contents of contracts. However, some of the consultants did recognize that the contracting process had had a beneficial impact upon certain hospital services.

The consultants' lack of concern over the standards may have been restricted to areas of the country where there was a lack of competition from alternative providers, as was the case for this multifund. Ham (1996) has suggested that one of the values of a contracting system is that providers have a stimulus to improve their performance because of the existence of other alternatives for purchasers. However, if this option is not present or very limited then Ham's idea of 'contestability' will not occur which may explain the consultants' ambivalence towards the quality standards in the first case study. A further reason why the local consultants did not feel threatened by competitive forces is that the fundholding GPs in the first case study were keen to support their local provider and were not prepared to use the internal market to damage local relationships; they were only prepared to 'shop around' at the margins. These findings relating to the relationships between fundholding GPs and providers concur well with Flynn and colleagues' (1996) findings in their study of community health service contracting.

The creation of GP fundholders had an important impact upon the intraprofessional relations of GPs and hospital consultants. The data from the first case study showed that most informants felt that the GP–hospital consultant relationship had become more equal. This greater degree of equality between the two branches of medicine was attributed to the fundholding scheme and the increased communication between these two groups, which fundholding was also credited with. The data suggest that as well as the GP gaining greater influence within the health service, primary care had also achieved a greater prominence. However, the hospital consultant was still considered an important figure by most informants, as many felt that their co-operation was still needed for changes to occur in hospital services. Many GPs felt that although they had a more equal relationship with hospital consultants they still sensed that consultants did not properly understand the world of general practice and they thought that many consultants still viewed them as 'failed consultants'.

The results from the smaller, second case study confirmed many of those from the larger, first case study. This confirmation in itself is significant as the informants at this stage were in a position to look back upon the impact of the 1991 NHS reforms as they had experienced eight years of these and were now entering a new set of reforms which they could also reflect upon. The impact that the fundholding scheme had had on both GPs and consultants was clear from this data. There was agreement among these informants that the scheme had raised the status of GPs vis-à-vis their consultant colleagues, and this has also been a finding of other studies into GP fundholding (Cowton and Drake, 1999; Dixon, Holland and Mays, 1998). There was also agreement among the informants that the fact that GP fundholders had control of budgets was the important determinant in the influence they had been able to exert over hospital consultants. An interesting adjunct to this perspective was the view that the status of consultants had decreased when compared to a hospital consultant 20 years ago. There was also some evidence to show that consultants had felt personally threatened in terms of their job security when some GP fundholders had started to move contracts away from this trust and they had reacted in partnership with the hospital management to recapture these contracts by launching a marketing exercise aimed at courting the local fundholding GPs. This suggests that the hospital consultants were ready to team up with the corporate rationalizers within their organization in order to maintain their resources (Alford, 1975, p. 209).

A strong message that arose from the data was that hospital consultants had had to increase their level of communication with the local GPs because the GPs had become purchasers. Formal mechanisms were set up where GPs and consultants could discuss how hospital services were organized, an area that had previously been outside GPs' sphere of influence. This was seen as a new development as communications between GPs and hospital consultants had previously centred almost exclusively upon clinical issues. GPs and consultants were now having discussions about how health services were organized and GPs were able to impart their perspectives on how services were managed and the changes that should be made. In other words the GP fundholders were successfully influencing the work of hospital consultants and restricting their power in certain areas, which can be said to be the goal of a corporate rationalizer (Alford, 1975, p. 209). The hospital consultants in the second case study felt that the GPs' perspectives had had a positive impact upon the quality of the services that they offered. The other positive outcome from the increased communication between GPs and consultants was that the informants felt that there was a better level of understanding of the problems that both sets of clinicians faced. The data from the first-round interviews in the first case study suggested that the GP fundholders were sometimes unrealistic in their demands of secondary care. However, the data from the second round of interviews in the first case study and the observations of the contract meetings indicate that after two years of contracting, the relationship between the multifund and the local trusts had matured into one that was based on mutual trust. The data in the first case study illustrate that prior to the abolition of the fundholding scheme the negotiations between the multifund and the local trust were increasingly based on co-operation rather than confrontation. This trend was also evident in the data from the second case study, which suggests that time had allowed the two sides to come to a better understanding and they could better appreciate each other's problems. Taken together the data suggest that the limitations of the internal market were recognized by both purchasers and providers and each side recognized the other's problems.

An issue that was more in evidence from the second case study data was that all the GPs recognized that the fundholding scheme had created inequalities between those patients who were registered with fundholding GPs and those who were not. Although the ex-fundholding GPs argued that the scheme had allowed them to offer their patients better services, it was recognized that another section of the population was not benefiting from this. However, the hospital consultants stated that the influence of GP fundholders had led them to provide better services and it was unlikely that the improved hospital services were only available to patients registered with fund-holding GPs. So the evidence suggests that although patients registered with fundholding GPs benefited the most, patients who were registered with non-fundholding GPs did also benefit from improved hospital services. This indicates that the fundholding GPs were able to have an influence over a wide area of hospital services rather than merely those that affected their practices. The managers in the second case study made an important point in relation to this. They expressed the view that the reason that GP fundholders were able to achieve changes in secondary care was that they had greater flexibility because they only purchased services at the margins. Health authorities that had been responsible for purchasing the bulk of the health services under the 1991 reforms could not be as flexible and these managers suggested that PCTs will also have to face this challenge. The data would suggest that it was the flexibility that GP fundholders enjoyed that allowed them to make changes in the provision of hospital services that larger primary care organizations would not have been able to achieve. This could suggest that PCTs may also fail to achieve the gains that some GPs made under the fundholding scheme, particularly if the predicted PCT mergers occur (Walshe *et al.*, 2004).

The issue of outreach clinics was a good example of the contested views of health service developments among the different stakeholders. Most GP informants, although not all, in the first case study felt that outreach clinics were a beneficial development as they represented a convenient and quick service for their patients and they credited the fundholding scheme with their growth. However, the hospital consultants in both case studies were far more sceptical of the benefits of these clinics. They felt that many patients who attended these clinics were not seeing the most appropriate consultant, as there was so much sub-specialization in modern medicine. The data from these two case studies were consistent with the results from other studies that have reported upon the limited value of outreach clinics in GP practices (Bailey, Black and Wilkin, 1994). The data on outreach clinics from the second case study provided an example of the inequity of such developments within the fundholding scheme.

5

HEALTH CARE QUALITY

INTRODUCTION

Having considered the impacts of the GP fundholding scheme both during its existence and following its demise, this chapter will focus on the data concerning the multifund's quality standards and the issue of health care quality more generally from both the first and second case study. Consequently, this chapter mainly draws upon the data from the first case study that had a substantial focus upon the quality standards that the multifund included within its outpatient contracts and their regulatory potential upon hospital consultants. By examining the implementation process of the quality standards, and hospital consultants', GPs' and other key stakeholders' perceptions of the standards, a picture will develop as to the impact the structural changes to the health service have had on the GP–hospital consultant relationship. The results from the survey part of the study will also be considered as these provide a greater level of comprehensiveness to the qualitative data, particularly that relating to the multifund's quality standards. The different perspectives of the informants upon the issue of health care quality from both the first and second case study will also be presented in order to examine how an informant's position within the health care system impacts upon these.

QUALITY STANDARDS

The first-round interviews in the first case study focused on the various informants' perspectives of the quality standards that the multifund had specified in their outpatient contracts. The informants were asked what they saw as the purpose of the standards, how important they felt they were and what their input into their derivation and implementation had been.

All of the GPs who were interviewed in the first case study felt that the setting of quality standards was an important issue. One stated that:

> . . . *the whole basis of wanting to improve primary and secondary health care is all tied up with quality standards and I think this is the very centre of fundholding.* (GP1)

Another multifund GP felt that the main aim of the standards was to bring all the hospital departments up to the level of the best:

> *I think the biggest expectation [of the quality standards] was that we would get more uniformity. That good directorates needn't get any better, but the bad ones might come into line.* (GP8)

Other GPs thought that quality standards were valuable because they provided targets that should be reached:

> *I think you've got to have some sort of yardstick, as it were, against which you can measure what you're doing* . . . (GP3)

Health service managers also felt that having standards was important as they provided explicit targets to aim for; they were seen as a possible way of measuring performance. A hospital manager who had previously worked in the private sector thought that written standards were important because

> . . . *you have a standard there and you either achieve that standard or you can't achieve that standard, if you can partly achieve that then you have the opportunity of totally achieving it in the future if you make changes or whatever. If you don't have written standards you have no way of measuring.* (M9)

A non-fundholding GP also agreed that quality standards were important but he also expressed a degree of caution. He felt the purpose of quality standards should be to

> . . . *set minimal standards rather than enforcing standards that perhaps some people would, or enforcing output that some people would find difficult to live up to.* [He warned that] . . . *those patients who need and want and expect a little more time and perhaps a more compassionate caring kind of approach, well,*

those consultants may no longer be there because they're too busy
sawing bones. (GP2)

This last comment illustrates the perceived regulatory potential
that over-demanding quality standards might have upon hospital
consultants.

When examining these quality standards it is important to analyse
how they were derived, as this process will affect their regulatory
impact. Although doubts have been expressed about the effectiveness
of non-participatory initiatives for standard-setting (Pollitt, 1993a),
many of the informants felt that that had been the multifund's
approach. The process was made up of three stages. First, discussions took place with other multifunds from outside the local area
about their experience of contracting and quality standards and
selecting the 'best' from these. Second, the medical manager (the lead
multifund GP who took an eight-months sabbatical to set up the
multifund) constructed other quality standards which he thought
would be appropriate from this particular multifund's point of view.
Last, there was a discussion among multifund GP representatives to
ratify all the standards that the medical manager had proposed. It
emerged from the interviews that the level of involvement and interest of the multifund GPs in fundholding in general and in the quality
standards in particular varied considerably. A multifund manager
made this point very well, when she stated that

> *There are GPs out there who I am sure have never even read*
> *the contracts. They're just filed in the practice, but there will be*
> *a fund rep. for every fund who has read them and has signed*
> *them on behalf of his fund, and has probably had a reasonable*
> *amount of input into what's contained in them but for the rest*
> *I don't think they probably know what the quality standards*
> *are.* (M7)

This may explain why the standards were developed in such a non-
participatory way. The quality standards were seen as a management
task by many of the GPs whose very reason, as has already been
illustrated in the previous chapter, for joining a multifund was to
hand over such obligations. The following multifund GP representative stated a widespread opinion among the multifund GPs who were
interviewed:

> *Well, I won't say they're not interested, they certainly don't know,*
> *I'm sure my partners haven't a clue about what the quality stand-*
> *ards in the contracts are . . . Most GPs are not terribly interested*

in the mechanics, they just want to get their patients in and get a good opinion. (GP7)

There seemed to be some difference of opinion among the inform-ants as to whose responsibility it was to monitor the standards, which could explain their low level of evaluation. On the one hand the GPs felt that evaluation was a management responsibility, which they as clinicians did not see as their role, while the managers thought that the GPs should play a major role in the evaluation of the quality standards because of some of the standards' clinical nature. There seemed to be obstacles to both groups' involvement. The multifund managers' priorities tended to be on the financial aspects of fundholding, leaving them little time to monitor the quality standards:

> *I think it would be fair to say that we haven't done anything seriously yet about monitoring or making sure that they [the quality standards] are adhered to ... our time has been wholly and utterly taken up by monitoring the financial side of things ...* (M7)

The data from the observations of the contract negotiations and evidence from other studies (Flynn, Williams and Pickard, 1996) also noted that these negotiations were dominated by financial con-cerns and any monitoring that was carried out centred on expenditure and activity rather than quality issues.

The problem of time was also cited by the GPs as a reason for not properly monitoring the quality standards. They felt that extra resources would have to be found if there was to be any meaningful monitoring of the standards:

> *I think really pressure of time to do all the other things we're trying to do ... Realistically at the moment it would be very difficult to do it [monitoring of the quality standards] with the resources we've got at the moment.* (GP8)

The evidence from the multifund informants suggests that although the idea of having quality standards in the outpatient contracts was viewed as important, the practicality of effectively implementing them was seen as a management task that they were unwilling to assume. Other practical problems such as a lack of time and resources meant that the multifund managers were also unable to effectively monitor the adherence of the quality standards.

Another important aspect in this area is the hospital informants' views of the quality standards. The issue of quality in its wider sense as opposed to the narrow aspect of the quality standards will be examined later in this chapter. However, it is worth noting here that a number of consultants in the first round of interviews raised the wider issue of quality in relation to the quality standards. Some of the consultant informants felt that the GPs' view of quality was rather superficial. This is how one hospital consultant caricatured the difference between a consultant's view of quality and that of a GP:

> *Whether you can survive it [the operation] or whether you're going to have the operation well done, that's what we [consultants] call quality of care, not how long you wait in the car park or whether the cup of tea's nice afterwards.* (C6)

These sentiments were echoed by another hospital consultant who stated that

> *I don't think they're [GPs] very interested at all. I don't think they're interested in clinical excellence at all. That's very controversial I guess, but I mean they're interested in getting them [patients] off their hands.* (C1)

The development of the quality standards was also characterized by a lack of involvement from staff at any of the multifund's provider units, that is, those who were expected to adhere to the standards that the multifund had developed. The lack of negotiation regarding the quality standards led the provider managers to feel that the standards being asked for were unreasonable. The hospital consultants, on the other hand, were not generally interested in the standards, to the extent that most of the consultants interviewed were unaware what standards the multifund had specified in their contracts, which was also reflected in the survey results that are discussed later in this chapter.

The contract director of a local trust summed up many of the views expressed by the hospital informants. He particularly resented the multifund's lack of flexibility when the contract specifications were under negotiation. He contrasted the health authority's attitude with that of the multifund:

> *With [the local health authority] we can negotiate because we know, we are dependent on them and they're dependent on us. That relationship should be there with GPs but we know that it isn't, and as I said before GPs are wielding their power quite crudely in certain instances. They slap them [the quality standards] on the*

table and say that's what we want. And we talk about the wording of it and they say no, no, no, that's what we want . . . I would say there's lots of discussion but I would say in reality there's little true negotiation. So what happens is, last year we signed the contracts, knowing we couldn't achieve them [the quality standards]. (M6)

The difference observed between the multifund's and the health authority's approach to contracting may be due to these two agencies' contrasting contracting responsibilities. The difference in approach may be due to the fact that fundholders were only responsible for contracting a narrow set of procedures while health authorities had to contract for the bulk of secondary care services, thus their flexibility in contract negotiations was quite different. This was an issue upon which both hospital clinicians and managers had a shared opinion as expressed by the following consultant, who felt that the multifund had to be prepared to arrive at a compromise about their quality standards, echoing what the contract director had said:

Well, I think there has been far too little of them [the trust] saying what they demand and because obviously the trust is at considerable risk to a multifund, you know a third of our income comes from them, so it's very difficult to say well bugger off I'm not actually interested, so one has to look at ways and I think, I mean I must say I think we should much more be saying well look I think we can go halfway towards that this year, and then do the other half next year, there's very little of that. (C1)

The hospital informants raised the issue of discharge summaries time after time in the interviews and it is a good example to use in order to explore their views of the multifund's quality standards. The contract director of the multifund's main provider unit felt that the GPs had made unrealistic demands on the hospital in the form of quality standards relating to discharge letters. The following comment reflects the early perception by providers of a somewhat bullish attitude on the part of GP fundholders:

For instance the GPs expect 100% of letters to be produced within a certain time . . . there's going to be an error rate, and that error rate has got to be accepted. But the GPs are currently pursuing 100%, rather than 95%. (M6)

A consultant informant pointed to the issue of discharge summaries as an example of the fact that they did not meet many of the multifund's quality standards. The following comment by a hospital consultant perhaps shows the result of imposed quality standards, or at least those that were perceived as being imposed on a provider:

I believe there is something in the contracts to say that discharge summaries should be provided within two weeks of the patient's discharge and we, like many other trusts, have been unable to come up to that standard on many occasions. (C4)

The impact of the quality standards on hospital clinicians' behaviour would seem to be minor, suggesting that their regulatory potential was not realized. The following consultant's view was a common one among those interviewed:

I mean it's very difficult to comment on [the multifund's] quality standards when I haven't seen them but you mention one of its contents, and we've talked about the discharge summary issue before and certainly having that in the contract, as far as I am concerned, doesn't seem to have altered what is actually delivered. (C2)

However, a multifund manager who argued that the rate and speed of discharge summaries had certainly improved since they had become fundholders contradicted the consultant's view:

Now, again that [discharge letters] was something the GPs had no clout to insist on but the minute we could withhold payment because the money was ours to control, hey presto they started to put systems in place to get us all these things. (M7)

Since hospital consultants are not actually involved in the administration of sending out the discharge letters to GPs the multifund manager's information is probably more reliable given that she was responsible for administering the receipt of these letters.

Another hospital consultant conceded that they did not manage to adhere to all the multifund's quality standards but they had prompted them to attempt to address the GPs' concerns. Again he gave the example of discharge summaries stating that

... at every meeting I've been to with GPs they talk about [discharge] summaries. And before we would say we can't do anything about it but now we are trying to do something about it, not very well but we are trying. (C1)

A multifund GP also felt that the quality standards contained in the outpatient contracts had had a negligible impact upon the service received by her patients:

> *I think the quality of the outpatient care is to me very much as it's always been. There are a constant stream of patients who come back into the surgery after being referred who haven't understood what's gone on at the hospital or have complaints about the length of time that they've been with the doctor for, the length of time they've had to wait.* (GP3)

However, another multifund GP had a more optimistic view of the impact of the quality standards, at least as far as discharge letters were concerned. He gave an example of the impact they had on a service:

> *Last year, in our first year of fundholding, there was a large number of, percentage of, letters that didn't come back from consultants following first outpatient appointment. Now because it was in the contract, the quality standards stipulated that we must receive our first admission letter by six weeks along with the invoice, otherwise no payment would be made. Now our provider lost a large amount of money. He simply wasn't paid. This year I guarantee you that that problem will not exist. So there is an example, quality standards are set, monitored and the quality was applied.* (GP1)

These data indicate that the quality standards had had an impact on issues such as discharge summaries but had had less of an impact on issues such as waiting times. This perhaps suggests that the monetary penalties connected to the late receipt of discharge summaries prompted the hospital management into action and the lack of penalties in other areas produced no change in the provider's behaviour. The data illustrate that the quality standards produced a behavioural change of hospital managers who put systems in place to improve the delivery of discharge summaries but had little regulatory impact upon hospital consultants. It is worth pointing out that it was the multifund managers who were responsible for linking the receipt of discharge summaries to contract payments. This shows that where the quality standards did have an impact it was between multifund and provider managers, in other words it was between the traditional corporate rationalizers and thus somewhat detached from the hospital consultants and the majority of GPs who acted as professional monopolizers, seeing these processes as managerial in nature.

The consultants did not think any of the quality standards were unacceptable in terms of their content, and the survey results also provide evidence of this. This may be because the quality standards that the multifund had selected did not attempt to lay down any clinical guidelines; they largely focused on organizational issues such as waiting times. Thus, the standards in the main impinged on the managers' sphere of work as opposed to that of the consultants, which perhaps explains the two groups' differing perceptions of the standards. The following consultant explains why he felt the quality standards did not impact on his work:

I would not be surprised if there was some requirement for me to see routine outpatients within a certain amount of time, again I'm not sure if having a contract would affect that because you know there is a waiting list and we try and get through the waiting list as fast as we can. (C4)

Perhaps an explanation for the consultants' lack of concern over the multifund's quality standards is that there were no penalties if the standards were not met or incentives for adhering to them. Furthermore, this research would suggest that due to a lack of monitoring and evaluation of the quality standards, on many occasions the multifund would be unaware whether the standards were being met or not. This is how one consultant saw it:

I have to say we don't achieve all the quality standards. Well again you see the problem is there's no real penalty at the end of the day when you haven't achieved it and if there was I guess we'd be in there, fighting much more at the beginning because that's what it should be. (C1)

Nonetheless, the way consultants practise will determine whether some of the quality standards are met or not. For example, the number of patients a consultant timetables in his/her outpatient clinic will influence the time individual patients are left waiting for their appointment in the outpatients' department and the size of the overall waiting list. On the issue of the multifund's current quality standards, the following consultant stated a widespread view among the consultant informants which was that if the multifund wanted them to be met then there were resource implications that he did not feel they recognized:

I think there's been a great thing of saying, particularly with GP fundholders, they very much say that they want this and this and that and that and this has to happen otherwise you know they're going to go elsewhere for their services, um but you can't do that, you may be able to, but you can't go on doing that, you can't say that your waiting lists have to come down but your activity remains the same, the sort of thing you know we don't want any waiting lists but you're doing too much work. You know there are limits there, I don't think that's recognised because they want the people to be seen now but who's going to pay for it? So I think obviously matching your resources to the activity you're looking for, also not just activity but the quality issues that are being pushed forward and, you know, those cost. (C1)

It is interesting to note that some GPs recognized that the failure to meet the quality standards was not the fault of consultants, but instead the blame rested on the trust management, illustrating the more traditional professional–management dynamic. The following multifund GP illustrates his medical collegiality by stating that he recognized that there were structural problems that consultants faced and he gave one example of these:

. . . quite often what we've found is that when quality standards have caused us a little concern, the consultants have wanted to do the very things that we wanted them to do but have been hindered by the policy of the trust. In practice for instance urology patients were having their routine operations cancelled time after time after time. The reason for this is that the urology patient bed status had been halved. (GP1)

COMMENT

This section of the data illustrates that there was a general agreement among the informants in the first case study that quality standards were important. The introduction of a set of quality standards enabled the multifund GPs to put into operation their demands for shorter waiting times and increased information from the hospital consultants. However, the fact that there had been little participation in the derivation of the standards both by the multifund GPs and the hospital consultants had affected their influence and their regulatory impact. One reason for the lack of participation in the derivation of standards on the part of the GPs may have been a consequence of the multifund's size. If this is correct it will have an important impact on primary care trusts which will in most cases be of a larger size

than this multifund. Although most of the GP informants saw quality standards as important they looked upon their operation as a
management function and were therefore in the main uninterested in
their mechanics. The quality standards were considered a corporate
rationalizing tool, and as such they tended to occupy the minds of
managers from both the multifund and the hospital trust (and then
only peripherally) rather than the doctors from both sides. The util-
ization of a set of quality standards is in itself significant despite
their limited success in achieving changes at the hospital level. The
evidence suggests that the GP fundholding scheme enabled some
GPs (in this case the medical manager of the multifund) to articulate
their quality requirements within a set of quality standards that can
be viewed as an essentially corporate rationalist framework. However, what is also clear from the data is that the majority of the
multifund GPs were uninvolved in the development and implementation of the quality standards. This evidence indicates that 'rank and
file' GPs were reluctant either to develop or implement the tools of
corporate rationalization in an attempt to regulate the work of
hospital consultants. The data suggest that many of the hospital
consultant informants were unaware of the exact contents of the
multifund's quality standards and even when they were it had not
substantially changed their behaviour in their view. However, the
data also illustrate that efforts had been made by the hospital trust
managers to improve the situation regarding discharge summaries,
which had resulted in improvements in their speed of dispatch, thus
responding to one of the multifund's demands. However, these
improvements were not the result of the GPs acting as corporate
rationalizers but rather the result of mechanisms being initiated by
the traditional corporate rationalizers in the shape of managers from
the multifund and the hospital trust.

DEFINING QUALITY

To examine the perspectives of quality more broadly the informants
in the first case study were asked what they considered to be a good-
quality health care service. Everyone agreed that delivering a high-
quality service was important. However, there were differences in
emphasis among the different health care professionals and all
the informants recognized the financial constraints on the service.
Informants acknowledged that the measurement of quality was difficult and multifaceted, it was not something that could be easily

defined, a point which has been reported in other studies (Hogarth-Scott and Wright, 1997). A non-fundholding GP argued that

> ... *the measurement of quality in general practice is almost certainly doomed to failure because there are so many different parameters by what you can measure quality ... I think it is almost impossible to measure the quality of an individual in general practice ... So really when you say, 'how do you measure quality in general practice?' I suppose my answer is pass.* (GP2)

Although the informants found it difficult to define a good quality service it was generally recognized that there was a growing emphasis within the NHS on delivering good-quality health care, an emphasis that has continued with the 1999 NHS reforms. This was a point that was made by the multifund medical manager:

> *I think there's far more emphasis on it now. I mean when I went into general practice basically GPs did what GPs do, full stop, end of story. Now, the catch phrases of 'clinical effectiveness', 'evidence based healthcare' are very much to the fore and I think after a while when you've been a GP for a while a lot of us feel that we want to know is what we're doing valuable or not?* (GP8)

However, GPs had a clearer idea of what they considered to be a good-quality hospital service – prompt and accurate consultations were sought from their hospital colleagues. As one GP stated:

> *Well I suppose it's one that answers questions you've asked and does it quite quickly and it doesn't keep on seeing them endlessly for no particular benefit.* (GP4)

The issue of outpatient waiting times, this is to say the time a patient has to wait between being referred by the GP to seeing the hospital consultant, was the most frequent one mentioned by the GPs, and this was confirmed in the results from the survey of health care professionals. The following GP expressed a very common view among the GP informants:

> *We have clinical meetings when we discuss a lot of clinical problems. One of our constant problems is obviously patients seen in a reasonable period of time ... The most important thing when you're sitting with a patient is to try to see if they need a hospital service, and it's only a very small proportion of the people we're seeing, they need it in a reasonable space of time and that's the constant aggravation of our general practice.* (GP7)

On the other hand, the hospital consultants argued that trying to keep waiting lists for outpatient appointments down without extra resources could have a negative impact on quality, demonstrating that the pursuit of one quality goal can clash with another. The following consultant expressed a widespread view among the hospital consultant informants:

> . . . *the trouble is then if you say right well actually we're not going to get more resources but you still have to keep within those parameters then you tend to see off people, more people quicker so that can affect your quality standards and if you're trying to stay within the same clinic time you've seen more people to keep your waiting list down then that clearly could compromise quality.* (C1)

The hospital consultants also found it difficult to articulate what they defined as good-quality health care. Components such as audit, good outcomes and professionalism were considered important, as the following comments made by three hospital consultant informants illustrate:

> . . . *an academic input and output and time made aside for appropriate audit and research is an essential ingredient.* (C2)

> *Well I think the major guiding force really is one's professionalism. One wants to deliver a service as high in quality as possible. So if there are any better ways of doing things than you've been used to then one should, one's professionalism really dictates that you should be adopting the new techniques.* (C4)

> *I suppose a good quality service would be achieved when you have a good clinical outcome as far as whatever medical condition the patient had with a satisfied patient at the end of it. Perhaps one has to add these days delivered in a relatively cost effective way.* (C3)

Although all the informants felt that the issues of quality and quality improvement were important, somewhat vague answers were given when they were asked about concrete quality initiatives. There was a mixture of formal and informal monitoring of quality carried out by most of the GPs and they felt that if their service was not of a high enough standard their patients were free to go elsewhere and this pressure would help maintain high standards. The comment from the following GP is a good illustration of a general view among the GP informants:

. . . all the time we are auditing our performance, for example if a patient goes out of the door and I know darned well that they're not happy with what I've done or said the next time I will or when I go home in the evening and the reason I don't sleep at night is all the time I'm auditing in my head what I've done wrong . . . I don't think we would be the successful practice that we are if it didn't have an impact. I mean there are a lot of very good practices locally and the very reason that we've got a successful practice is that if we didn't audit and try and improve what we did we would soon find ourselves with a falling list of patients. (GP2)

Quality was a rarely discussed issue during the contract negotiations that were observed and in those reported by informants, as one contract accountant stated:

The quality side of it is an area we are not so up front on I have to say . . . The GP fundholders don't tend, they really sort of monitor the quality by exception shall we say . . . Certainly from the fundholding purchasers, they're not demanding quality issues. (M5)

The hospital consultants felt that the monitoring of quality that is generally carried out by fundholding GPs tended to be of a quantitative nature and did not address quality issues that they felt were important. The following consultant informant illustrates this point of view:

. . . whereas in fact all they're interested in is, is he a nice guy or he arrives and he sees them in our own clinic within a month. That is as far as I can see the only quality standard that we're talking about. Or we send him up to the clinic and he doesn't have to wait half an hour to be seen. Now when I've got my cancer, yes I understand that it's important not to be kept waiting for a long time in out-patients. I understand that the guy I see ought to be nice but frankly that's bottom of the pile in terms of something that may or may not kill me. (C6)

However, this same consultant did make the point that non-clinical quality was important and hospital consultants may have overlooked this area in the past:

. . . [surgeons] were blinded by those clinical standards and they weren't sufficiently concerned about waiting times, access to hospital car parking, communications with the GPs which are very important but you know, I think we tended to disregard those almost completely and it was right and proper but I say most of

that's come about through the Patients Charter and not through the contracting process. (C6)

The multifund medical manager did recognize that the issue of quality had become a rather crude counting exercise and that it was important to look at issues such as clinical outcomes:

I'm interested in looking harder at what we're doing, the outcomes really of what we're doing. I think a lot of it that's been done up until now has been a budget balancing exercise and a counting numbers exercise, you know, how many people have had out-patient procedures, in-patient procedures, day case procedures? What I'm really interested in is the outcomes of those procedures . . . (GP8)

The data from the first case study demonstrated how GPs' and hospital consultants' views of quality differed at least in terms of emphasis, and this point also emerged in the second case study. The data from the second case study also show that the principal quality concern for GPs was the length of waiting times, particularly the amount of time their patients had to wait to see hospital consultants; this is how one GP expressed a widespread concern among the PCG GP informants:

I think if I am a patient, when I am ill I should see the doctor early as possible. So the patient should not wait that long to see them [the consultant]. That is number one. (GPiii)

However, a hospital consultant felt that this was a simplistic way to view quality. His view was similar to those that were expressed by hospital consultants in the first case study:

. . . a lot of GPs have only been bothered about how quickly a patient's been seen, they're not actually bothered about who's seen them and what the outcome was. (Ci)

Both hospital consultants and GPs recognized that the quality of care in general practice was patchy and this was something that would have to be tackled:

. . . you've got some wonderful practices with some wonderful buildings and highly skilled, highly knowledgeable practitioners working together, and you've got others that are still in 1948. And I think that difference can't be sustained for very much longer. (GPiv)

The new primary care structures may be able to tackle these wide variations of quality between practices. Another study reported that this was an area that PCGs were beginning to address as part of their clinical governance agenda (Baeza and Campbell, 2001).

The quality of GP referrals has often been a complaint about primary care from hospital consultants and this was an issue raised by consultant informants. They often judged the quality of the GPs by the referrals that they received, as this consultant informant pointed out:

> . . . *some of the referrals we get from some practices are just not up to scratch. And that is in spite of literally ten years of talking to them around guidelines and protocols.* (Ciii)

Overall the consultant informants felt that quality was an issue that had been pushed up the health policy agenda. They all saw this as a good development as long as the final arbiter of quality was a clinician:

> *I don't see why anyone would manage outside that protocol scenario. Equally, I think it should be the clinician, and it is the clinicians, if you like, in his or her gift, to do outside that in consultation, provided there is a very sound clinical reason for doing so. I think the days of, 'This is the way I've done it for twenty years,' is history.* (Ciii)

Consultants felt that new policies that had been introduced aimed at improving the quality of health services such as clinical governance were an important development and that such mechanisms would be used to regulate their work:

> . . . *we're much more answerable, our quality, obviously, is pinning people down, protocols, we've got to agree on what a standardised management should be. So clinical governance obviously is important. And that's going to regulate performance.* (Cv)

Consultants also felt that patients themselves will play a more significant role in the delivery of health services in the future and become a more powerful force within the health service as a whole. One hospital consultant felt that in the future patients would become increasingly better informed and as a consequence will wish to become more involved in their treatment:

> *I mean in the next few years patients are going to be incredibly well informed, because they're going to be getting all the information*

they want off the Internet, plus locally supplied information will improve, and we'll end up with some much more empowered patients. (Ci)

COMMENT

This section illustrates that health professionals consider quality to be an important aspect of their work and that the issue of quality had become more central within the health service as a whole. However, the informants found it difficult to articulate what constituted a good-quality health service. The data illustrate that there was a contested view of quality among GPs and hospital consultants. The second case study helped to confirm the findings regarding the different perspectives on quality held by consultants and GPs. The GPs' priorities of shorter waiting times and increased information from the hospital consultants were reflected in the multifund's quality standards, which the multifund attempted to implement within their outpatient contracts with limited success, as the data illustrate. There was evidence from these informants that the issue of quality had achieved a greater importance within the health service and had perhaps become more structured; for example, the consultant informants felt that the new policy of clinical governance will have a regulating effect upon them. As a whole, the data suggest that health care quality is becoming increasingly bureaucratic in nature and is being framed in corporate rationalist terms both at the macro level of government with their introduction of clinical governance and at the micro level of a GP multifund including a set of quality standards in their outpatient contracts. The patient and professional surveys carried out in the first case study help to provide further evidence on the issue of quality and quality standards and these results will now be examined.

THE SURVEY STAGE

The two questionnaires conducted in the first case study investigated the views of both users and health care professionals on the awareness, acceptability and importance of the quality standards used by the multifund in its outpatient contracts (see the Appendix for the response rates and further methodological information on the surveys). The aim of presenting data from the two surveys of users' and health care professionals' views on the awareness, acceptability and importance of the quality standards is to shed further light on how the various groups' perspectives might be similar or different with regard to quality. The survey results help to add a greater level of comprehensiveness to the interview-based evidence. The results from the survey of health care professionals will be considered first.

When the health care professionals' survey results were taken as a whole it showed that two-fifths of those who responded were not aware of the multifund's quality standards. Furthermore, 80 per cent of those who answered stated that they had not been consulted about the standards. The evidence from the qualitative interviews in the first case study on the importance of quality standards was also supported by the survey results, which showed that 89 per cent of the respondents felt that quality standards were either important or very important.

The survey results were even more revealing when the responses were split up by professional group. The results presented in the graphs below confirm the picture that emerged from the qualitative evidence from the first round of interviews in the first case study, showing that it was not only the hospital consultants who were unaware of the standards but only just over half of the multifund GP respondents were aware of their own multifund's quality standards (Graph 5.1).

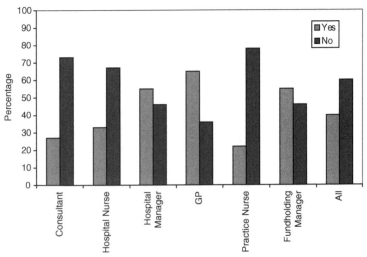

Are you aware of the multifund's quality standards?

Graph 5.1   The level of awareness of the multifund's quality standards

The results are even starker when it comes to the degree of consultation about the quality standards, where less than 5 per cent of hospital consultants and only just over half of the multifund GPs reported that they had been consulted (Graph 5.2).

However, as Graph 5.3 shows there was ambivalence, particularly among hospital consultants and multifund GPs, as to whether the quality standards should include clinical issues; these views were also evident in the data from the interviews that will be reported in the following chapter. The other professional groups felt that this may be an appropriate development.

The acceptability of many of the multifund's standards was high across all the groups of respondents. Where there were marked variations in perspectives it was usually between hospital doctors and general practitioners and additionally between those on the purchasing and providing sides. These differences are illustrated by Graphs 5.4 and 5.5, which asked about the various groups' acceptability of two quality standards that are contained in the multifund's outpatient contracts.

It is clear from Graphs 5.4 and 5.5 that there is quite a marked dichotomy in views in terms of the acceptability of these two particular standards between the health care professionals from the

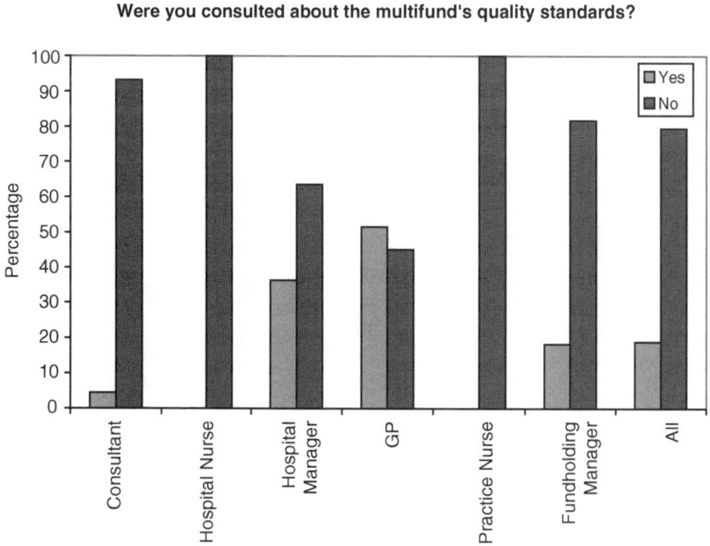

Were you consulted about the multifund's quality standards?

Graph 5.2 Degree of consultation of the multifund's quality standards

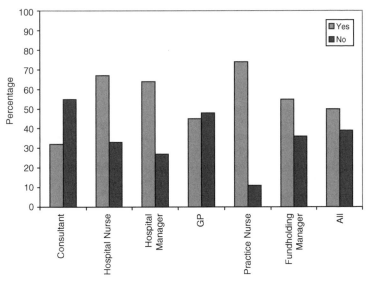

Graph 5.3   Should the multifund's quality standards cover clinical issues?

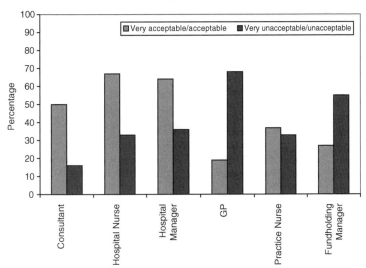

Graph 5.4   Acceptability of a standard on outpatient appointment waiting times

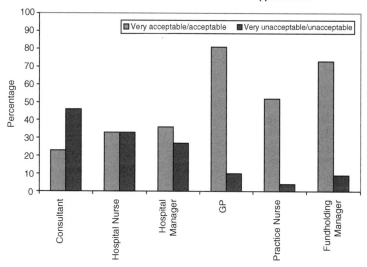

The number of follow-ups following an operation is to be a maximum of 2, except for cancers. The outpatient doctor will inform the GP when a further appointment is necessary. Lack of comment can be taken as consent for a further appointment.

Graph 5.5 Acceptability of a standard stating the maximum number of follow-ups

provider trust (represented by the hospital consultants, hospital nurses and hospital managers) and those from the purchaser side (represented by the multifund GPs, practice nurses and fundholding managers). There was little evidence of any overall difference in perspective between the managers and health care professionals; the differences were instead between purchasers and providers, that is to say the differences were intraprofessional rather than interprofessional. They were not, therefore, an Alfordian difference between corporate rationalizers and professional monopolizers, which is perhaps a reflection of the importance and influence of the structural separation between primary and secondary care in the NHS. The differences were particularly evident within what could be seen as the traditional professional monopolizers, that is to say between the hospital consultants and the multifund GPs. These differences were further illustrated by the answers given to the open-ended questions asked in the survey. In answer to an open question, which asked which issues quality standards should cover, over a third of the hospital consultants who answered stated that the quality of care given in the outpatient department should be addressed; issues such as clinical effectiveness and outcomes were also mentioned by the hospital consultants. On the other hand only four of the GPs who answered mentioned these issues. In contrast, their main concern was the length of waiting times for their patients' outpatient appointments. Respondents from the provider side also mentioned that quality standards had resource implications. Lastly, nearly a quarter of the consultants who responded stated that quality standards should be set for the referrals that GPs make to the outpatient department.

Similarly hospital doctors and users were in disagreement, or put another way, users had more in common with general practitioners. This was well illustrated in relation to the general issue of waiting times. The only two standards that registered any notable level of unacceptability among the users were concerned with waiting times. The satisfaction rates of the outpatient services among those users who responded were very high. However, the lowest satisfaction rates were recorded for the waiting times between seeing their GP and their outpatient attendance and the amount of time they had to wait in the outpatient department before their consultation – nearly a fifth of the respondents felt these were either very unacceptable or unacceptable. It is important to note that the issue of waiting times produced the highest rates of dissatisfaction among users, which is the same issue that GPs considered as important in their survey.

The survey of professionals found that the level of awareness of the multifund's quality standards was low among them as a whole and particularly low among consultants. Although there was a high overall level of acceptance of most of the quality standards, these levels differed between the professional groups. Hospital consultants and GPs disagreed on the importance of certain quality standards; there was also evidence of a dichotomy of opinion on some standards between general practice and hospital staff, particularly between hospital consultants and GPs. The survey of recent users of the outpatient department showed that the standards were highly acceptable to them and that the users reported high levels of satisfaction with most aspects of the outpatient service. Users reported some dissatisfaction with the waiting times for outpatient appointments and the waiting time once in the outpatient department.

SUMMARY

The multifund GPs had a paradoxical view of the quality standards; on the one hand most of them saw them as an important element within the contracts, while on the other hand they viewed them as an uninteresting management function that they did not consider part of a GP's job, thus not engaging in a corporate rationalizer-type function. The multifund GPs' lack of engagement in the mechanics of the standards may have been a consequence of their adoption process or conversely, the general lack of GP interest in the standards may have led to them not participating in the adoption process. The empirical evidence, both qualitative and quantitative, indicates that there was a low level of involvement by the majority of the multifund GPs and the hospital staff in this process. The non-participatory method of developing the multifund's quality standards resulted in disenfranchising most of the GPs from them, which ended up with a set of quality standards that were not monitored or evaluated by most of the multifund GPs. A national survey of purchaser contracts found that not only were monitoring methods vague but there was wide variety in the complexity and detail with which quality standards had been approached (Maheswaran and Appleby, 1992). The reason that many of the GPs were not involved in the implementation of the quality standards was that they did not consider it as part of their job and were happy to leave it to the medical manager, who in turn tended to devote his or her limited time to the financial aspects of the contracts. This evidence suggests that the majority of the GPs did not see their role as being involved in what they perceived to be the management activities of implementing and monitoring a set of quality standards. In other words most of the multifund GPs were not keen to utilize the somewhat bureaucratic tools involved in corporate rationalization.

The evidence also shows that there was a lack of consultation and negotiation about the quality standards with the providers' clinicians and managers. The contract managers were dissatisfied with the multifund's approach, that is the perceived lack of negotiation and flexibility, because it resulted in signing off on standards that the hospital could not meet in their entirety. Flynn and colleagues (1996) identified a similar situation when they reported that contracts were being signed before the work on specifications had been completed. This poses a management problem and there is also evidence to suggest that a more negotiated and co-operative approach between trusts, fundholders and health authorities can lead to improvements in patient care (Moore and Dalziel, 1993).

The evidence from the first case study would seem to suggest that the GPs' perceived gain in influence has not been at the expense of the consultants, as the hospital consultants appeared indifferent to the quality standards and the manner in which they were imposed. The consultants' attitude towards the standards is perhaps a reflection of the lack of evaluation and monitoring of the standards. Another contributing factor may be the lack of penalties for non-compliance or rewards for achieving the quality standards, thus failing to provide any incentives for them to modify their behaviour in line with the specified standards.

Hospital consultants thought that many of the standards were acceptable, although their level of acceptability and importance of some of the standards differed from that of GPs. The survey and the interview data from both case studies provided evidence that consultants' and GPs' views of quality differed in emphasis. From a GP's point of view it was important that their patients who needed to see a specialist should see one soon; on the other hand, consultants considered the outcome of such consultations as the most important issue and felt that a speedier throughput without extra resources could have a detrimental impact on outcomes. However, it was not clear from the data whose definition of quality was dominant; what was clear was that the GP fundholding scheme via the contracting process had allowed GPs to articulate their quality priorities to hospital consultants in a way that had not been available to them previously. Most informants felt that providing higher quality care and achieving the quality standards had resource implications that were not always recognized; other researchers have also reported this (Appleby, Smith, Ranade, Little and Robinson, 1994).

The data from both case studies illustrated the difference in perspectives between GPs and hospital consultants on the concept of quality. A contested view of quality emerged: hospital consultants tended to prioritize outcomes while GPs were concerned about waiting times. The survey results tended to indicate that GPs' quality concerns resonated well with those of patients, suggesting that at least in this respect GPs were good proxies for patients. There was also evidence from the data that the issue of quality had achieved a greater importance within the health service in recent years. Both GPs and hospital consultants perceived general practice to be of variable quality, which is an issue that will need to be tackled if greater collaboration between primary and secondary care is to develop in the future.

6

TRANSFORMING INTRAPROFESSIONAL RELATIONS?

INTRODUCTION

This chapter considers the empirical evidence concerning the relationship between GPs and hospital consultants more directly and examines how the changing primary care structures over the past ten years have affected this. The importance of the GP–hospital consultant relationship within the health service will also be highlighted. This chapter will focus upon the data from the first multifund case study relating to the GP–hospital consultant relationship during the era of the fundholding scheme and the influence the multifund's quality standards had upon the work of hospital consultants in particular and hospital services more generally. Alford's (1975) structural interests typology will be used in order to understand how and to what extent the intraprofessional relations between GPs and hospital consultants have been transformed. The data from the second primary care group (PCG) case study sheds light on the likely impact the new primary care organizations will have upon the GP–hospital consultant relationship.

THE GP–HOSPITAL CONSULTANT RELATIONSHIP

The multifund's quality standards were seen as a good way to investigate the important GP–hospital consultant relationship as they were situated at this professional interface. Although the standards were largely about organizational issues, it was the consultants who were ultimately responsible for delivering them, as it was they who were responsible for the patient while in the outpatient department.

In order for the GPs to challenge the hospital consultants' behaviour they need to behave like corporate rationalizers who are interested in extending their control into the hospital arena and the key hospital professionals that work there (Alford, 1975, p. 192). For this reason it is important to examine the hospital consultants' perspectives of the multifund's quality standards as the GPs were attempting to use these to influence the behaviour of hospital consultants. A family health services authority (FHSA) manager summed up the importance of consultants very well in relation to achieving change when he stated that

> *... at the end of the day you will make faster progress if the consultant wants it, and if the consultant doesn't want it you will have a lot of trouble making progress, so the consultant is a key factor.* (M3)

The importance of hospital consultants and their dominant role within the health care system was illustrated by the experience of one non-multifund fundholding GP who explained how changes in services could be blocked by hospital consultants, who as professional monopolists are largely satisfied with the status quo (Alford, 1975, p. 195). He gave the example of outreach clinics:

> *Well I suppose consultants coming out to practices. I mean that's a big thing and I'm not sure that would have happened without fundholding really. Again, I think certain consultants don't really like to do that. We wanted to bring a dermatologist in house but we weren't able to find anyone who wanted to do it really.* (GP4)

This example indicates both the possibilities and the limitations of the previous fundholding scheme.

The FHSA manager also made the point that the GP–consultant discussion is important because they are both part of the medical profession:

> *The reason I think the consultant and GP dialogue is so important is because they talk the same language.* (M3)

When examining the intraprofessional relations of GPs and hospital consultants it is important to consider the informants' views upon the extension of quality standards into clinical rather than largely process-type areas. The quality standards that were used by the multifund did not in any way attempt to lay down guidelines for clinical procedures. Most of those who mentioned this issue did not consider the inclusion of clinical quality standards to be appropriate now but some felt these would certainly be introduced in the future. A health authority manager felt that the setting of clinical quality standards would take time due to the sensitive nature of this issue. He thought that

> *In some way that is a far more long term process, because you're really starting to get into the issues around clinical responsibility and the independence of the practitioner and all those kind of issues . . . [that] needs a much softer approach . . .* (M2)

Hospital consultants felt that clinical guidelines would become more widespread but they were keen to emphasize the importance of personal clinical experience within medical care. Various hospital consultants echoed the statement below made by a consultant informant:

> *I can see clinical protocols coming but clinical autonomy is difficult to argue against . . . Individual patients need individual treatments and you only get a feel for that by personal experience.* (C3)

GP informants felt that evidence-based practice was important and should become more prevalent:

> *I think we've always shied away from protocols . . . I think it's a very good potential development, yes, take evidence-based medicine, that's the classic, people should be doing much more evidence-based medicine because with some of the things we deal with in medicine are witchcraft.* (GP5)

However, there was also the recognition from GPs that this was a sensitive issue and developments in this area would have to be made cautiously. This GP acknowledged the fact that if he referred a patient it was to obtain a hospital consultant's opinion that he or she had to be free to make and so he felt that formulating collaborative guidelines was the way forward:

> *We can influence that to an extent [thresholds for surgery] but there is a lot of discomfort about doing that, because, as a GP if you are asking for a specialist opinion you presumably regard that as higher opinion otherwise you wouldn't be asking for it, then to say well actually I disagree with you, I don't want that doing, is potentially confrontational. If you can work together on guidelines that's the best sort.* (GP8)

All of the GPs who were interviewed felt that there was a more equitable relationship between them and consultants, which had not always been the case. The following multifund GP expressed a common view among the GPs regarding the new GP–consultant relationship:

> *They've [the consultants] certainly realised that their livelihood depends upon attracting our patients and our patients' money and they've had to listen . . . it's now much more of a two-way street, instead of us sending the patients up to them for their opinion for them to look after, it's more a matter of we lend them a patient for them to give an opinion and give the patient back to us. And they accept that we can sometimes give them quite a lot of information and help them as well. Oh I think the power has gone very much towards general practice.* (GP5)

This perception of a new, more equitable relationship between GPs and hospital consultants, as well as being attributed directly to the fundholding scheme was also ascribed to the increased communication between the two groups which the scheme had spawned. The following GP expressed his surprise when he observed how consultants were now far more ready to attend meetings with GPs:

> *. . . we had a couple of meetings when we invited consultants to come over, it was a very strange feeling for the GPs really, you know, the mass, they nearly all came . . . to listen to GPs, what the GPs were up to.* (GP7)

The increased communication that the fundholding scheme had prompted had led to a better understanding of each other's situation, as this GP explained:

> *. . . we are getting to know our consultant colleagues far better because of the interaction between the consortium and the trusts . . . we're actually getting to meet them far more regularly, finding out what their problems are. They are learning to trust us and feel that we are their allies . . . There's a lot more respect I think for the consultants now from the GP point of view because we can see how hard they are working, how much pressure there is on them and their departments.* (GP1)

Most of the GPs felt that it was the fundholding scheme that had decisively shifted the balance of power from the consultants to the GPs, as the same multifund GP argued:

> *They've [the consultants] suddenly found that they are totally and completely dependent upon referrals whereas before we referred*

we were totally dependent on them calling our patients and I think it's completely shifted, totally. (GP1)

A health authority manager also felt that structurally the GP practice had achieved a far greater prominence within the health system, stating that

I think probably the most significant thing that has changed through contracting has been the potential shift away from the hospital, which has been very much the power base to the GP surgery being the power base. (M2)

The following multifund GP neatly summed up how she perceived the new GP–hospital consultant relationship:

. . . the Christmas cards now come from the consultants to the GPs rather than the other way round. (GP3)

Although most multifund GPs felt that they had gained power vis-à-vis the hospital consultants they still thought that the relationship should be seen as one of partnership rather than a fight for power. These opinions illustrate the paradox in the GP–hospital consultant relationship, where the GP recognizes a professional alliance with the hospital consultants but at the same time appreciates the need to challenge some of their practices.

However, a hospital manager felt that there were only relatively few GPs who were using their fundholding status to confront the hospital consultants:

. . . there are some of the cavalier GPs out there who want to own the waiting lists and tell these damn consultants who they'll operate on, when they'll operate, etc., etc. But they are very few and far between. (M6)

The hospital consultant informants recognized the potential leverage that fundholding GPs had within the internal market but they also saw that the GPs' potential power to move contracts and thus threaten consultants was limited in reality. The following consultant explained how moving contracts at the margins could destabilize other hospital services, so this power would have to be used sensibly:

It certainly seems that they [GP fundholders] have purchasing power, but I would hope that they would use that responsibly because if they decide to take substantial business away from their local hospital in one sphere, then that may well have a knock-on effect on other activities within that hospital, activities which they, the fundholders would very much like to see maintained within that hospital so they would have to take a very balanced decision really. (C4)

The hospital consultants also highlighted another constraint on GPs' potential power of moving contracts between hospitals. The following senior consultant informant, who had a lot of contact with consultants in other parts of the country because of his involvement in medical politics at the national level, explained that outside London the possibilities for moving contracts from one hospital to another were limited in many specialties:

> . . . *in the early days when people were flexing their muscles and getting behind the barricades, there was always this threat that if you don't get my patient sorted out within two months, I'm going to send them somewhere else . . . then you're in a very disadvantageous position, if they decided to pull the plug on you and contract with another hospital. This has been obviously highlighted in London where there are plenty of other opportunities around the corner . . . whereas down here you have relatively less flexibility . . . In other words the GPs have got nowhere else to go if they want to threaten my specialty.* (C5)

These examples suggest that the 1991 internal market had a rather limited impact in non-metropolitan areas of the country due to the lack of alternative providers.

The consultant informants also felt that fundholding had given the GPs more power within the health system but many of them felt that their power gain was not at the expense of the consultant, particularly in day-to-day terms, as this consultant explained:

> *I suppose in terms of political power, quite clearly the GPs have got much more than they had and the balance has gone that way. I'm not sure that it affects us at all day-to-day. Because largely they are still dependent on us but although I mean they have the opportunity of sending cold surgery to Timbuktu, all the acute work happens here and basically not many patients want to go elsewhere. So there's quite a lot of bluster and bluff but I don't think we have a perception that we're being threatened by the GPs.* (C1)

This same consultant explained why it was difficult for a GP to threaten a consultant's power base, illustrating the deep-rooted nature of their dominance within the health care system:

. . . I think that it's very difficult from their (a GP) point of view
if I say as a specialist this should happen. How on earth can they
turn round and say it shouldn't? (C1)

There was also a general feeling among the hospital consultants that
the power of the medical profession as a whole was generally on the
wane due to the bureaucratic demands of their jobs, and as part of
this trend the all-powerful consultant was a thing of the past, as this
consultant argued:

I am sure there are individuals that feel very powerful but I don't
think they are, the GPs are overawed by it, they're pretty depressed
by all this bureaucracy, the consultants are overwhelmed by bureau-
cracy, nobody feels omnipotent and empowered and autocratic and
I'll do what I want, it isn't like that and it hasn't been like that in
practice for a very long time. (C6)

COMMENT

The data illustrate the central importance of the GP–hospital consultant relationship within the NHS. The data indicate that both GPs
and consultants felt that clinical guidelines and protocols would
become more prevalent within the NHS, although informants felt
that advances in this field should proceed with caution and in a
shared manner. The development of National Service Frameworks
(NSFs) at a national level is a manifestation of this policy trend.
There is evidence that although the hospital consultant is still an
important figure within the health service, GPs have managed to
develop a more equitable relationship with their hospital consultant
colleagues. This new relationship has resulted, in part, from increased
communication between the two branches of medicine that the GP
fundholding scheme had promoted. There was evidence that the contracting mechanism within the fundholding scheme had given the
GPs the potential to extend their control into the hospital environment and hospital consultants' activities. The result of these new
intraprofessional relationships may further extend the role and
importance of primary care within the health service, making it a
more effective challenge to the hospital. I will now turn to examine
data relating to the influence the multifund had on the hospital sector
that was derived from the second round of interviews in the first case
study.

INFLUENCING SECONDARY CARE

The second-round interviews in the first case study investigated whether the multifund's quality standards had had an impact on outpatient services. In other words, were GPs able to use the quality standards as a tool to control the behaviour of the hospital consultants and thus behave like corporate rationalizers (Alford, 1975, p. 201)? GPs and multifund managers felt that they had probably only had a marginal impact on the service, as this comment by a multifund GP illustrates:

> . . . *I can't honestly say I've seen a vast improvement from patients coming back . . . I think if you looked at figures it probably is happening but actually sitting in a chair I don't notice it.* (GP6)

A hospital contract manager felt that many of the multifund's quality standards were implicitly worked to, as they were part of a doctor's professionalism. The following example illustrates how corporate rationalizers (here the contract manager) sometimes ally themselves with professional monopolists (hospital consultants) within their own organization in order to increase their legitimacy (Alford, 1975, p. 209):

> *They [the consultants] don't need a GP to write on a piece of paper, work to the standards to which you were trained and work every single day of your life and have morals etc, etc. So there's an actual base level anyway which you need to assume is consistent with GPs' expectations but it's implied because everything's now explicit in terms of documentation and openness, there's an implication that quality should be written and documented and worked to a standard when in fact that's probably happening already.* (M6)

The above quote illustrates the move from implicit standards that are based upon high trust relationships to explicit codified standards that are based upon written documentation, a move towards what Power (1997) refers to as an 'audit society'. It is significant that this codified relationship is developing within the medical profession, between GPs and hospital consultants rather than between managers and clinicians, thus GPs are utilizing the tools of corporate rationalization.

Informants from the provider and purchaser sides, doctors as well as managers, recognized that some of the quality standards were not attainable within the current health care resources – all the informants would have agreed with the following comment made by the multi-fund manager:

> *At the end of the day also, when you put all these wonderful quality standards in and yet you can't manage to give the hospital back their financial expectation and you're asking them to accept a contract that's valued at less than they really needed, how much can you demand that they follow all the quality standards on every occasion because every time you introduce something and they say the funding isn't there for it the Health Authority won't fund it. We haven't got the growth monies to be able to put that sort of thing in place.* (M7)

This illustrates how factors such as finance limited the influence that the quality standards could have upon hospital services. It shows how some of the changes that the GPs wanted to make to hospital services through the quality standards were not considered possible within the prevailing financial environment, which meant that the control that GPs could exert on the work of hospital consultants was limited. However, it should be recognized that the perceived financial constraints may have been a tactic that both hospital managers and hospital consultants used to limit what they were willing to provide to the multifund and a way of maintaining the status quo. The effectiveness of this tactic, if that is what it was, upon the multifund is evident in the multifund manager's quote above.

These second-round interviews were carried out between 12 and 18 months after those of the first round of the first case study. In the intervening time the perceptions of contracting had changed among the informants; the relationship between the multifund and the local trust had become more established and the confrontational undercurrents had disappeared as this multifund manager explained:

> *I mean two or three years ago it probably wouldn't have been quite like that. It's matured an awful lot . . . The distrust, if that's what it was, and the concern about each other has gone. We each know that we put our figures on the table. It's what we've got. There is no more. Do what's best that both sides can do with the situation.* (M7)

The multifund's medical manager had come to understand the realities of contracting. There was a greater appreciation on the part of the multifund of the impact on the hospital of moving contracts from one provider to another, as the medical manager explained:

I think our relationship with the local hospital has matured. Initially it seemed quite simple. We were purchasers. They were providers. The more you learn, the more complex you realise the relationship is. There's a knock-on effect of everything you do and in order to help one speciality in the hospital you may actually disadvantage another. So you may find that there are winners and losers within even one hospital and that is difficult for the consultants to understand, I think, sometimes. (GP8)

Informants were also asked whether or not they felt that their work had become more regulated and whether an instrument such as quality standards could be used in a regulatory way. There was a feeling among the informants that there was a greater degree of regulation in the NHS generally; it was recognized that some regulation was probably necessary, although both GPs and hospital consultants saw dangers in an over-regulated service. These two comments by a hospital consultant and then a multifund GP illustrate their argument:

I think a certain amount of it [regulation] is important because ultimately it's a public service and we have to be accountable to the public via the politicians, managers and administration . . . but I think there is a distinct danger of this approach being too heavy handed and if it's taken to an extreme, and if we become over-regulated I think the professionalism will suffer. (C4)

Unless you're the clinician on the spot you cannot really dictate how long someone should stay in hospital. I don't think you can anyway. I would feel very nervous about dictating to a consultant colleague, you know, that you're actually keeping people in too long, stop doing it. I don't think that's our role. (GP8)

These comments illustrate the importance placed upon the idea of professionalism by the hospital consultants, which was a concept mentioned by several of the consultant informants. On the other hand the GP informant recognized the boundaries between the responsibilities of GPs and hospital consultants and felt uneasy about dictating the work of hospital consultants.

However, the following multifund GP was quite clear about the influence over consultants he felt he had due to the fact that he was a fundholder:

There has been a heart change from the specialists' point of view because they would never have been sensitive to what general practitioners wanted for their patients. Had it not been for the fact that the money follows the patient it would never have happened in a million years . . . I think only the financial carrot and stick made it change . . . they would not have made the change happen had it not been for the clout of being able to be fundholders. (GP1)

The following GP explains how he felt that as fundholders they had been able to reduce waiting times for certain specialties but that their initial successes were already beginning to fade, which perhaps reflects the transitory nature of some of the improvements to hospital services that GP fundholders achieved:

I mean the eyes waiting list was almost a year I think before fundholding. It came right down and there's still quite a bit of a wait and the same with dermatology but again the waiting lists are better than they were but they're starting to creep up again. (GP4)

The hospital consultant informants all felt that their influence had decreased within the health service; this is an observation that was also made by the consultant informants in the second case study. The following consultant explained why he felt their power within the health service had declined over the past two decades:

We're more interfered with . . . when I was first a consultant 21 years ago the consultants were in charge. I mean, you know, they called the shots. As they said it, it happened. Now, unfortunately that was an enormous responsibility and it was not always discharged responsibly and very reasonably people got anxious with the system and it wanted improving. It has now been improved so people now monitor us and interfere with us. (C6)

There was a view among both consultants and GPs that there was a need for a better understanding between them. This is an issue that also came out clearly in the second case study of a PCG. The following GP informant explained what many GPs thought the reason for the lack of understanding on the part of hospital consultants was:

. . . until consultants have got to spend some time in general practice in the same way that general practitioners have got to spend time in hospitals, consultants would never properly understand what goes on in general practice. Perhaps now that the fundholders are able to meet with consultants and hospital managers and let them know what happens in general practice then perhaps even those consultants who've never been in general practice are beginning to understand that we are not failed consultants. We are not

high-grade mental defectives as they have taken us to be and that in fact there are problems that are quite special and specific to general practice just like there are problems that are quite special and specific to hospital units so I'm not saying that GPs should influence the way that consultants work but what I'm saying is that the consultants should understand what the special problems with general practice are. (GP2)

The data from the second case study indicated that the advent of PCGs might allow more health care to be undertaken within the primary care sector. However, the movement of health care services from secondary to primary care preceded the creation of PCGs as the data illustrate. The multifund medical manager explained how one of his objectives behind setting up the multifund had been to enable GPs to move more health care from the hospital into the GP surgery:

The traditional primary/secondary divide is something that's being examined by lots of people and we are, I hope, playing our part in that as well. The idea of trying to change the way in which clinical care is delivered across primary and secondary care is one of my main interests of coming into this. For instance more work in-house in general practitioners' surgery buildings, more work in the cottage hospitals, outreach out-patient clinics and more direct access services into the hospital rather than going on traditional out-patient appointment first, then the investigation, then out-patient appointment afterwards. So there's an economy in terms of use of NHS resources and a faster delivery from the patient's point of view, also trying to influence the number of . . . unnecessary follow-up out-patients appointments which occur perhaps usually through junior staff who haven't got the experience to say we'll discharge the patient, hanging onto them and is rolling on and on and on which again clogs up out-patients, increases the waiting times and doesn't really do any good for the patient if there's no need for it. (GP8)

The following two multifund GPs explained how GPs were already carrying out work within primary care that was once performed in the hospital:

. . . we're now actually doing a lot of work that the consultants were doing before, freeing them up to concentrate on the really ill people in hospital and that's quite a proud thought really because then you're helping consultants to really utilise their time in a

more effective way. That is providing they're not on the golf course! (GP1)

. . . but again more and more work is being pushed into the primary care. We see that too with patients being discharged from hospital and receiving treatment in the community which previously might have been dealt with in hospital . . . (GP3)

These examples illustrate the growing importance of the GP surgery within the health care system. This is a development that could have a profound impact upon the future delivery of health services and is something that the current government is actively encouraging (Department of Health, 2002). However, the movement of work from secondary into primary care will have an impact upon GPs' workload, which is something that needs to be addressed if this shift is to continue and it may act as a brake to further developments in this area. The following multifund GP explained that although carrying out more work in his surgery might be beneficial for both him and his patients, changes in the GPs' work patterns may need to occur for this to continue, which again illustrates some of the constraints that exist to the increasing influence GPs can have upon the service:

. . . we do much more in primary care than we did when I started. That is a good development, those facilities can go on expanding, there's still stuff that goes to hospital that doesn't need to . . . I think that if you have smaller list sizes, the more GPs the smaller list sizes, you could certainly do even more in primary care than you do now, OK I'll do that here, brilliant, rather than trekking over to some clinic but that means that I've got to put 15 minutes of minor op time into my day, which I do because I enjoy doing it and get a small fee for it, but that can't go on endlessly. (GP7)

COMMENT

The data in this section suggest that GPs have been able to influence certain areas of secondary care; however, their influence has been limited and may have been of a short-term nature under the fundholding scheme. Many informants saw the perceived lack of resources within the service as an insurmountable barrier that prevented the GPs from achieving their desired changes to hospital services. The NHS still suffers from the perception of a resource-scarce organization despite its recent period of financial growth. There was evidence in the second round of interviews that the relationship between the multifund and the local trusts had matured and developed into one based more on co-operation than confrontation. Although most informants felt that the GP–hospital consultant relationship had improved because of the fundholding scheme there were still some GPs who felt that consultants needed a better understanding of the issues that GPs faced in order for this relationship to become truly equal. Many informants felt this was because medical education lagged behind medical practice, making education an important issue within the health policy process. The data also illustrate that primary care as a whole is gaining greater prominence within the health system with certain hospital services being provided by GPs in their surgeries; however, this trend is constrained by the limit on the extra workload GPs are prepared to undertake, which is a particular problem when one considers the current GP shortage. There was evidence that the GPs were exhibiting corporate rationalizing tendencies but in common with the traditional corporate rationalizers (that is, health service managers) they were experiencing the somewhat in-built limits to their influence within the service.

COLLABORATION

A greater degree of collaboration within the NHS was one of the professed aims of the health policies the new Labour administration introduced – an NHS that would be based on collaboration rather than competition (Light, 1999; North, Lupton and Khan, 1999; Chisholm, 1998). The second PCG case study examined how the hospital consultant–GP relationship had been changed by the first Labour health reforms and the issue of collaboration within the health service was explored. There was a widespread view among the informants that consultants and GPs had gained a better appreciation of each other's work and the problems that each of them encountered. This greater degree of understanding, which was emerging towards the end of the fundholding scheme, had been achieved by the increased communication between GPs and hospital consultants which had been a side effect of the scheme. There was evidence that the 'them and us' attitude between consultants and GPs that had been present in the earlier days of fundholding had softened. This is how one consultant described the impact of the increased level of communication between GPs and consultants:

I think consultants have got more respect for GPs than before. I think because we get together so much more and people can understand a little bit more about what each other's role is and what life is like for each other, so I think there's more mutual understanding and more partnership. You know, there's less polarisation, and it's a more mature relationship. And I think something that hopefully has changed forever is the clinicians, be they primary or secondary care, recognise that they need to talk to each other face to face. (Ci)

However, this same consultant did not regard this greater degree of communication as a development that will continue without continued effort; he felt that it was something that could disappear if it was not worked at:

. . . where I think an organisation like this can still go wrong is that the assumption that good communication and good co-ordination between GPs and consultants will just naturally continue, because I think it needs to be more of a managed process . . . (Ci)

These comments illustrate that if the communication between the two is to continue then resources in terms of management and time need to be devoted to its maintenance. Further research will be needed to determine whether the collaborations that have begun to develop will continue and what impact this will have upon the NHS as a whole.

The first case study established that the fundholding scheme caused some initial conflicts between GPs and consultants. However, the second case study illustrates how the greater degree of communication between both sets of clinicians had bound the two sides of the profession together, perhaps restraining the development of GPs' corporate rationalizer-type characteristics and highlighting the common interests they share with hospital consultants as professional monopolists (Alford, 1975, p. 197). As one consultant said:

Let us talk to the GPs. Let us sit round the table, clinician to clinician, agree what we want and then let the managers facilitate what the clinicians think is best for the patient . . . we found that when we were clinician to clinician, our priorities were exactly the same, which was good. (Ciii)

This indicates the hospital consultant's view that there are common interests that exist between GPs and hospital consultants and the perception that managers should merely facilitate this relationship between like-minded professionals.

This same consultant used the example of the development of guidelines between primary and secondary care to illustrate how the two branches of medicine could collaborate to a greater extent in the future and promote a professional understanding:

> *I would like to think that guidelines and protocols are developed in consultation between GPs and the consultants, keeping all higher professional bodies' views and guidelines.* (Ciii)

One GP informant insisted that the important dialogue was the one between primary and secondary care clinicians, with managers acting purely as the facilitators, thus echoing the views of the hospital consultant informants. He gave the example of the orthopaedic department that had needed an extra consultant and how with the GPs' support the consultants had succeeded in obtaining the trust management's agreement to release the resources that were needed to employ the additional consultant: a good example of GPs and hospital consultants working in concert to achieve shared professional aims. At the same time this GP felt that the consultants sometimes saw the GPs as the enemy when they suggested that more services should be moved into primary care. This GP gave the example of outpatient clinics: he felt that there was no need for them to be run from within the hospital where there were large overheads; in his view these clinics could be provided more cheaply either in GP practices or in two or three sites in the community. This GP stated that consultants argued against this, protesting that such a development would have an effect on the teaching of juniors, but in his view if services are being carried out in the community then that is where the education of juniors should be taking place. He felt that such restructuring of services would threaten hospital consultants who will therefore be resistant to these fundamental changes. This GP informant felt that:

> *These developments could mean that consultants lose their empires. Medical education should follow service development and not the other way round as at present.* (GPii)

The comments made by this GP illustrate the importance medical education has on the organization of a health care system, stressing the fact that medical education needs to keep up with medical practice. They also illustrate that there are still important differences between hospital consultants and GPs on how health services should be structured and where they should be located. Where the aspirations of GPs and hospital consultants coincided they would work together, using their professional influence to achieve their joint aims. However, on other issues GPs were prepared to challenge hospital consultants in order to change the status quo. It is possible that continued collaboration between secondary and primary care clinicians will enable services to be restructured so as to offer the best outcome for patients. However, the perceived differences of opinion reveal the different structural interests of GPs and consultants, illustrating that many of the current structures within the NHS favour hospital consultants, who are therefore keen to preserve them while GPs are eager to challenge them.

It is possible that a greater degree of collaboration between the two branches of medicine may in the future lead to a greater degree of trust between consultants and GPs – something that is needed if GPs are to take a more central role in the total care of their patients. One GP described how the development of direct access to hospital services by GPs had resulted in shorter waiting lists for certain hospital services. He gave the example of direct GP access to magnetic resonance imaging (MRI) scans. GPs could now write to the consultants requesting an MRI scan for their patient so that when the consultant does see them they will be in possession of the scan results. The GP felt that these arrangements would lead to faster access for patients by freeing up more outpatient appointment times. Another example given by this GP was of having fewer follow-ups in secondary care by passing the management of patients on to GPs at an earlier stage, thus freeing up consultants to see patients who were on the waiting list. However, these procedures are still developing as not all the GP practices have these arrangements with the local trust in place. These developments need changes in administration as well as consultants changing their practice in order to allow GPs to take more responsibility for their patients; it relies on hospital consultants having a greater degree of trust in their GP colleagues, but it also entails a releasing of control on the part of consultants. The GP informant who described these examples felt that these developments had occurred as a result of the increased co-operation between GPs and consultants.

However, one consultant illustrated how the level of trust that is needed for the greater development of GP direct access to hospital services was perhaps still absent on the part of some consultants, arguing that

> *. . . you could have every GP requesting a same day CT scan or MRI, you know, you'd need to build up the training, the protocols,*

tremendous amount of trust before you could sort of open your services up in that way. (Cv)

It is interesting that this consultant feels that he owns these services, which indicates a reluctance to reform the current structures that help to maintain their dominance within the health care system.

COMMENT

The data indicate that collaboration is not a neutral activity but is closely related to issues of power. It is not just a matter of whether collaboration between GPs and hospital consultants occurs; it is the nature of this collaboration that is important. The data suggest that although there was a lot of rhetoric about collaboration from the hospital consultant informants there was a feeling among the GP informants that the collaboration that hospital consultants were willing to engage in had definite limits. These limits tended to be related to resources, particularly in terms of hospital services that could be directly accessed by GPs such as certain diagnostic instruments. However, another thread that runs through the theme of collaboration is that both GP and hospital consultant informants had a perception that they had common interests that derived from their shared vision as professionals and that managers were clearly outside this arena, illustrating the classic doctor (professional monopolizer)–manager (corporate rationalizer) divide.

THE IMPACT OF PRIMARY CARE GROUPS

At the time of the data-gathering for the second case study, PCGs had only been in place for a year so informants were asked what impact they felt these new structures would have on the service as a whole. Some informants felt that even at this early stage certain changes had already occurred as a result of the abolition of the fundholding scheme for GPs and their subsequent absorption into PCGs. This is how one ex-GP fundholder and current PCG board member saw the situation:

I think certainly 50 per cent of patients were members of fund-holding practices and got a very good deal under the last administration and 50 per cent didn't. Now no one's getting a good deal, and everyone's just been getting a very mediocre treatment . . . It's been levelled down to pre-fundholding. (GPiv)

However, this same GP informant felt that not all their powers had been lost after the abolition of the GP fundholding scheme. He explained how some had been retained within the new PCG structure:

GPs still have some power at PCG level, rather than at individual level. So I think the individual level power they may have had as fundholders, that's gone. But you're quite right, there's still that residual stuff, you still get good discharge summaries and that sort of thing. (GPiv)

This indicates that although the abolition of fundholding blunted the power of those individual GPs who belonged to fundholding practices many of the gains that had been achieved by GPs overall, such as quicker receipt of discharge summaries, had continued. Another GP informant who was also on the PCG board felt that the new structures had retained the advantages associated with the fundholding scheme and done away with many of the drawbacks, but this process would inevitably take time to develop, and some patients may experience some initial deterioration in services as the transition occurred. He felt that consultants had to realize that primary care could deliver many services more cheaply and more conveniently for patients. However, these changes in service development had needed the fundholding scheme to occur first and would not have taken place without the foundation of fundholding in primary care.

The GP informant who had not previously been a fundholder welcomed the fact that now all the GPs within the PCG were treated more equally. He also felt that being part of a PCG had increased the communication between GPs:

The fundholders, they look only at their practice, not worried about what's happening next door. But now the PCG is concerned with all seventeen practices . . . The GPs are talking to each other, which we didn't do before. (GPiii)

Another GP informant felt that the creation of PCGs had had a negative impact on his professional autonomy. He felt that being part of a PCG had decreased his personal level of independence compared to that enjoyed under the fundholding scheme, pointing to his restricted freedom to refer his patients to the hospital he wished:

When we were fundholding, we had a bit of independence, but now everything has to be done through the PCG ... there's the odd thing I wanted to send down to Trust A ... I could use them if I wanted. Now I can't. I've got Trust X and Trust Y and that's it ... the freedom of my work has been compromised. (GPi)

This quote illustrates that although the influence of the GP population as a whole had been preserved despite the abolition of the fundholding scheme, individual GPs' freedoms were perhaps more constrained within the new corporate structures that PCGs represented.

There was a feeling among the GPs who were not on the PCG board that they did not know what the PCG was doing for them. This GP informant explained his concerns:

I've had two newsletters or something, and the newsletters I don't understand. I don't know what they're doing on my behalf. (GPi)

This indicates that the PCG structures were suffering from the same internal communication and involvement problems that were evident in the multifund structure and that they would only increase in PCTs.

A GP who was a member of the PCG board also recognized that GPs would probably not yet have experienced any changes due to the PCG structure, and the changes that patients were experiencing had so far been negative:

I don't know that many GPs in the field would have noticed a great difference with the PCG. All they will have noticed is that their patients are waiting longer to have various treatments. (GPiv)

While most of the GP informants felt that the demise of the GP fundholding scheme and the creation of PCGs would diminish the GPs' powers and freedoms, the hospital consultants saw the creation of PCGs as giving greater power to GPs within the NHS. This was because in the consultants' view PCGs, and then PCTs, would be the commissioners of all secondary care services. One consultant saw the creation of PCGs in this light and felt that this may have its problems:

... now it's everything, and all secondary care, so the GPs are going to have ultimate power ... I think there's nothing wrong in principle with primary care really calling the shots and configuring a type of service that the consumer wants, the patient wants, you know. The worry is that power is falling into the hands of people with vested interests and everything else. Well I mean that GPs may purchase services that suit them rather than consulting with the patients to see what service they want. (Cv)

A senior hospital consultant agreed that the new primary care structures will enhance the power of GPs and that many of the changes achieved by fundholders would be pushed further forward by the new primary care structures.

Another hospital consultant also recognized the potential problems the new structures might have on him as a professional, again echoing the ideas of professionalism expressed by consultants in the first case study. He felt that the kind of procedures that would be carried out in secondary care in the future might impact on the work he did and his role as a hospital specialist:

> *I suspect they [GPs] will dictate as to exactly what sort of services they want for their patients. And I have no problem with that . . . Professionals within the service need to develop and need to have a career structure, and they need to see themselves flourish within the working environment. And giving a silly example, if one PCT says that in a certain speciality they just need bog-standard, for example, ENT, grommets, tonsils and adenoids and nothing else, whereas the hospital side of things said, 'Okay, we provide that service, but in addition we want to do the big cancer stuff. We're a cancer centre, we want to do the cancer stuff.'* (Ciii)

Another senior consultant also felt that there might be a conflict of interests with the new primary care structures due to the fact that PCTs will be both commissioners and providers of health care services:

> *I think there is a potential conflict of interest in being a provider and a commissioner . . . I don't think they should be regulating our internal structure. They would have ultimately, presumably, the power to commission somewhere else if they didn't like the quality . . . So I think they have to be aware of the global picture and what they want for, not just their own patients, or even the PCT's patients, but for the economy's or health community's.* (Cii)

However, this consultant did at the same time recognize the potential merits of the new primary care structures:

> *. . . provided it's a reasonably mature organisation, then probably working with PCTs will be better than working with a whole disparate group of fundholders. But it will depend on, I think, how they evolve really.* (Cii)

Another consultant hoped that in the future PCTs and the GPs

within them would want to work in collaboration with hospital consultants in order to solve problems:

> *So my hope is that the PCTs or the GPs out there will get into*
> *dialogue with the secondary care providers like us and say, 'Look,*
> *this is our problem, this is not your problem or, you know, one side*
> *or the other. It's a collective thing. Let's have a collective*
> *approach.'* (Ciii)

However, collaboration between primary and secondary care will
only occur if communication between the clinicians on both sides
continues, as the previous section showed. The data from the second
case study illustrate that the links between the new PCGs and the
trusts are at a very early stage and require time and commitment in
order to succeed. A consultant who had the task of linking up with a
local PCG explained his view of the problem:

> *We invite GPs but we rarely ever get them here. They probably say*
> *the same thing about us, because I'm supposed to be a link with the*
> *PCG, but I think it's a couple of months since I've been able to go*
> *to any of their meetings. So time is a really big problem.* (Cv)

It has been suggested by certain commentators that in terms of
cost effectiveness more clinical work should be carried out in primary care (Light, 1999). Both GPs and hospital consultant informants agreed that more procedures had to be carried out in primary
care so that there could be faster access to hospital services. One
senior consultant put it quite simply:

> *And we need to unclutter the hospitals of what shouldn't really*
> *need to be there. The only way you do that is to do more in primary*
> *care.* (Cii)

Another hospital consultant shared this view, giving examples of
what care should and should not be carried out in the hospital
setting in the future:

> *The future, I think, of secondary care, in my view, is providing that*
> *category of service which is not possible in the primary care set-*
> *ting, and perhaps consultants like me doing the heavy, technically*
> *demanding, difficult work that cannot be done out there . . . I*
> *hardly do a vasectomy in this hospital any more. The GPs out*
> *there are doing it. They liaise with us. If there are patients who*
> *they're not happy with, we get them, we do them. And there are*
> *other procedures that are shifting. And that is fantastic.* (Ciii)

A GP informant very much agreed with the fact that more could and was being done in the primary care setting. He stated that GPs were referring some cases to other GPs like himself instead of referring their patients to consultants. It was the new flexibilities present in the PCG structures that had allowed this GP to carry out more minor operations in his surgery. Before PCGs he could only be funded to carry out five minor operations a month, now the PCG could contract him to carry out more:

> *... because I am a surgeon, I've got referrals from other GPs ... instead of writing to the hospital, now the GPs are writing directly to another GP ... so we can decide where to send the patient, either to a GP or a specialist.* (GPiii)

A health authority manager also felt that carrying out more work within primary care was the way PCGs were going to proceed in the future in order to reduce waiting lists for hospital services:

> *... in terms of engagement with the PCGs around waiting lists, there is much greater opportunity for them to say, 'We can do this in primary care. This doesn't need to be on a waiting list within the secondary care sector. Let's deliver it.'* (Mii)

A GP who was a member of the PCG board felt that both GPs and consultants needed to change their work practices so that more could be done in primary care, illustrating how significant the GP–hospital consultant relationship is:

> *GPs could manage more of their patients' needs if consultants developed management plans and this would again free up secondary care time. Consultants must be more ready to let go. GPs also need to be ready to let go so that they can take on the extra work. They need to pass on work to their practice nurses, such as blood pressure monitoring and the management of diabetics and asthma.* (GPii)

One of the consequences of the new primary care structures has been that GPs have had to adapt to the corporate structure of PCGs, which is quite different to their traditional individual or practice viewpoint. Other studies have reported that this shift in approach might prove a problem for some GPs (North, Lupton and Khan, 1999). This GP informant, a PCG board member, described the shift that GPs had to make:

> *... part of the education that we've been bringing down to practices*

is to say, 'Look, actually you're no longer an individual prescriber running your own business. No matter how you like it, or not like it, we're now in a systemic model of health care delivery, and you are a member of [the outer London] PCG, and what you do has an impact on the PCG because the PCG can't overspend on its budget.' (GPiv)

The above quote also illustrates the self-policing role that will be occurring among GPs within PCGs, which may lead to a process of restratification within the GP population, leading to further heterogeneity within the medical profession. A PCG manager also recognized the difficulty of changing GPs' focus from their individual practice to the larger PCG and then PCT:

I think the problem we've got is moving the GPs from their practice bias to the corporate bias. (Miii)

This shift in focus within primary care was also noted by a senior hospital consultant who felt that primary care needed to catch up with secondary care in terms of governance:

. . . whatever the ills of the hospital service, there has been a degree of regulation, mostly informal but latterly more formal of practice, and more of a need to conform. I think general practice has been very much unregulated, both financially and clinically in governance terms. (Cii)

A senior trust manager warned that managing GPs was a very difficult task, jokingly stating that:

. . . managing consultants in a hospital is like herding cats, but managing GPs is like teaching cats synchronised swimming! It's that hard. (Mi)

A health authority manager warned against PCGs trying to do too much too soon; she felt that PCGs needed to focus on sorting themselves out internally before attempting to reconfigure secondary care services:

. . . it's very easy for the PCGs currently to get pulled into the interest in the secondary care sector and not into sorting out the primary care sector. (Mii)

The second round of interviews in the first case study established that a greater degree of collaboration was occurring between GP fundholders and hospital trusts. The data from the second case study illustrate that this trend is continuing and perhaps being promoted further within the new health service structures. However, the data also indicate that this collaboration needs investment in order to continue. The data also suggest that in spite of this increased collaboration there was still more to be done in order to develop a greater degree of trust between GPs and hospital consultants that would allow more health care services to be provided within primary care.

SUMMARY

The data presented in this chapter illustrate the importance of the GP–hospital consultant relationship within the NHS. There was evidence that this relationship was of a more equitable nature than it had been prior to the 1991 reforms and there was a greater level and quality of communication between primary and secondary care doctors. The data suggest that this may not be so much a redistribution of power between the two branches of medicine as a levelling down of influence among a weakened medical profession. GPs recognized that there should be limits to their influence over hospital consultants and there was a general reluctance among the informants to develop clinical standards in any unilateral way. However, GPs did not feel that the world had totally transformed since the introduction of the GP fundholding scheme; they still sensed a certain lack of understanding of general practice by the hospital consultants. Some GPs attributed this lack of understanding to the fact that medical education still focused on hospital medicine at the expense of general practice, which is in itself a reflection of the dominance of hospital medicine and hospital consultants. General practice will have to challenge the medical education system so that it reflects modern medical practice rather than lagging behind medical practice, as is currently the case.

Ex-GP fundholders in the second case study felt that the abolition of the fundholding scheme had led to the deterioration of the services they could offer to patients and to a decrease in their influence within the health service as a whole. However, these same GPs also felt that within the new primary care structures they had managed to retain some of the powers that GP fundholders had enjoyed. Some GPs felt that the new PCG structures would manage to retain the advantages of fundholding without the inequalities that had been perceived to be present in the scheme. However, it was felt that this situation would take time to develop and the fundholding scheme had been a necessary precursor. The GPs who were not on the PCG board had a limited awareness of the activities of the PCG; this could be because the PCG was still in a developmental stage. The consultant informants all felt that the new primary care structures would further enhance the position of GPs. They recognized that PCGs would be responsible for commissioning all health services and so would place GPs in a powerful position. The consultants expressed some fears about the possible conflicts between the commissioning and providing responsibilities of PCGs. The results also suggest that the links between the PCG and the trust were weak; this may prove an obstacle to building on the increased communication between primary and secondary care clinicians that had developed during the GP fundholding era.

The data suggest that PCGs and now PCTs will want to carry out more functions within primary care, thus freeing up hospitals for those services that could not be performed in the primary care setting. For this to become a reality a culture change on the part of both hospital consultants and GPs was needed. Consultants will have to develop a greater trust of their GP colleagues and relinquish their control over certain services so that GPs are free to order a wider range of hospital tests for their patients prior to their referral and transferring more of the aftercare of patients to GPs, thus reducing the number of hospital outpatient follow-ups that patients currently experience. However, hospital consultants may be unwilling to reform these structures which enable them to maintain a dominant position within the present health care system and it remains to be seen how successful GPs will be in forcing change upon them. GPs also face new challenges as they will have to be prepared to take on more responsibilities for their patients and they will also have to adapt to the new corporate nature of PCTs that enables referrals to occur among GPs. GPs will increasingly have to face the paradox of having an enhanced influence over health services at a group level but at the same time many 'rank and file' GPs will experience reduced levels of individual autonomy.

7

INTRAPROFESSIONAL FUTURES

INTRODUCTION

This final chapter will review the key features of the study as a whole before going on to discuss the implications of the findings from the two case studies that were presented in the preceding three chapters. Specifically, this chapter will discuss to what extent, if at all, general practitioners (GPs) are displaying, in Alford's terms, corporate rationalizer-type tendencies as a consequence of the health reforms that occurred during the 1990s. The evidence from the first case study will be examined in order to assess to what extent the measures contained within the 1991 National Health Service (NHS) reforms enabled GPs to challenge their hospital consultant colleagues. The permanence of any changes and the possible impacts of the 1999 primary care structures upon the GP–hospital consultant relations will then be discussed in the light of the evidence from the second case study of a primary care group (PCG). The chapter will end by discussing the merits of deploying Alford's (1975) theory of structural interests in order to analyse how the intraprofessional relations of GPs and hospital consultants within the English NHS have been changed by the 1991 and 1999 NHS reforms.

AN OVERVIEW

Chapter 1 charted how the medical profession in general had managed to amass its influence during the past century and a half. It also illustrated how various health policies had affected general practice and hospital doctors in different ways and how the two sections of the profession reacted to reforms in varying modes. Although the fortunes of these two branches of the medical profession waxed and waned during the twentieth century, it was the hospital consultants who were in the ascendant. Their position was further strengthened with the creation of the NHS when Bevan was forced to make various concessions to hospital consultants in order to gain their support. After an expansion in the welfare state in general in the 1950s and 1960s, the fiscal crisis in the 1970s prompted the state to pursue cost containment policies towards public services such as the NHS. Cost containment and the pursuit of quality were to remain persistent health policy themes for successive governments during the 1980s and 1990s. The quest for better quality health services was to be increasingly used by governments in their attempts to regulate the still powerful medical profession.

Chapter 2 critically reviewed the health reforms of the 1980s and 1990s, illustrating how successive policy-makers have expended a great deal of energy upon the NHS in general and the medical profession in particular. Many of these efforts have had a negligible impact upon an organization and a profession that have proved to be largely resistant to change. The 1980s' social policy agenda was dominated by the expansion of managerialism into the public services. The introduction of general management in particular, which replaced consensus management, represented a major defeat for hospital consultants (Harrison and Ahmad, 2000). General practice was subjected to the basic tenets of managerialism with the creation of Family Health Service Authorities (FHSAs) and the imposition of the 1990 GP contract (Warwicker, 1998). Although on the eve of the major 1991 NHS reforms the medical profession's autonomy and dominance as a whole had declined when compared to their situation 20 years previously, this decline had not been the same for both sections of the profession. Hospital consultants were subjected to indirect challenges to their authority in the form of general management while general practice had both indirect challenges in the form of FHSAs and much more direct ones such as the imposition of a highly directive contract (Warwicker, 1998). This difference of approach to the two branches of the medical profession is just one illustration of the relative dominance of hospital consultants when compared to their GP colleagues prior to the implementation of the 1991 reforms. Although both branches of the medical profession have been through crests and troughs throughout their history, as Chapter 1 discussed, hospital consultants have always been regarded as superior to GPs (Harrison and Ahmad, 2000; Mahmood, 2001).

Chapter 3 introduced the issue of power and how it can be approached from various ideological and theoretical viewpoints. It was argued that a structural interests approach such as the one articulated by Alford (1975) is a helpful framework by which one can analyse health policy. However, it was also recognized that there were certain weaknesses in this framework, particularly Alford's view of a relatively homogeneous medical profession. The medical profession cannot be viewed as a relatively homogeneous body made up of practitioners with similar points of view who will always act in a unified way when their autonomy is threatened (Williams, 2001; Cho, 2000; Lewis and Considine, 1999). In the light of this discussion, Alford's conception of structural interests was used in order to examine whether what Alford (1975, p.192–3) calls the *internal contradictions* within the dominant structural interest have resulted in more of a long-term realignment of structural interests where GPs are now the agents of corporate rationalization who are now challenging the hospital consultants who remain the professional monopolizers and continue to defend the status quo that serves their interests.

Alford's structural interests model was explained in Chapter 3 and the empirical work set out in Chapters 4, 5 and 6 sought to investigate whether GPs could be usefully viewed as the new corporate rationalizers following the 1991 and 1999 NHS reforms. In particular, the two case studies examined whether GPs, through policies such as fundholding and then within PCGs, could be characterized as the new corporate rationalizers within the medical profession. Elston (1991) argued that the continued pressure from the centre to contain costs by attempting to limit the medical profession's freedom to spend resources

> . . . *may be invoked primarily through new forms of institutionalised professional control over members rather than through managerial fiat. It may turn out that it is the 'corporate rationalizers'* **within** *the profession who are in the ascendant.* (p. 76, emphasis in the original)

Elston (1991) did not elaborate further upon this proposition. North (1995) in a similar vein has suggested that fundholding GPs could be seen as both corporate rationalizers and professional monopolizers, although again she did not expand on this. In a later article North and Peckham (2001) argued that as fundholders GPs were *being incorporated as fledgling corporate rationalizers* (p. 429). It is these propositions that this empirical study set out to investigate more fully.

At the end of Chapter 3 Alford's theory of structural interests was used to examine the impact of the health reforms that occurred during the 1980s and 1990s. It was suggested that as well as attempting to strengthen the hand of the traditional corporate rationalizers, in the shape of health service managers, the 1991 reforms also gave GPs, by way of the fundholding scheme, the opportunity to influence the provision of hospital services. The creation of an internal market placed the two branches of medicine in two clearly defined camps: GPs as fundholders became the purchasers and hospital consultants had become the providers of health services. This view of two separate camps emerging within health care was reflected in the survey of health professionals that was carried out in the first case study site (Graphs 5.4 and 5.5 in Chapter 5). The results from this survey illustrated that on many issues there was a definite provider–purchaser split rather than, perhaps a more expected, doctor–manager split (Baeza and Calnan, 1999). Introducing such a clear split between the two branches of the profession could potentially destabilize the dominance of the medical profession as a whole within the health care system and create a fracture between the GPs, who were now the purchasers of health care (as well as maintaining their primary care provider function), and the hospital consultant providers.

The structural changes that have occurred to the health care system in England have been profound and the empirical evidence contained in Chapters 4, 5 and 6 provides a basis on which to examine their possible impact upon the GP–hospital consultant relationship. First, Chapter 4 examined the informants' perspectives of the fundholding scheme both during its existence and then after its demise by using data from both case studies. Chapter 5 explored the idea of health care quality; this was largely comprised of the interview and survey data from the first case study in relation to the multifund's quality standards. The final empirical Chapter 6 concerned itself mainly with examining how the creation of primary care groups might alter GP–hospital consultant relations. It is the conclusions that can be made from these data to which this chapter will now turn.

GPs AS REGULATORS?

It has been argued that the important change that the 1991 reforms introduced was the contracting mechanism that GPs in fundholding practices could potentially use to influence secondary care in general and hospital consultants in particular. The data in Chapter 4 illustrated that one of the reasons the GPs gave for joining the fund-holding scheme was that they felt they could use the contracting process to influence the secondary care sector. The multifund GP informants in the first case study were not eager first or second wave entrants into the fundholding scheme; they were somewhat reluctant fourth wave fundholders who felt that having control over their practice budget would give them the opportunity to have some bearing on secondary care services. The data illustrated how the GP informants considered the fundholding scheme as being the vehicle by which they could have a greater degree of influence upon hospital services. Although influencing hospital services may have been the original aim of primary care-led commissioning schemes such as GP fundholding, studies have reported that these commissioners tended, instead, to focus on developing primary care services (Smith and Barnes, 2000). Concentrating upon primary care services may have been a response to the GPs' frustrated attempts effectively to influence secondary care services. The inclination to concentrate on the development of primary care, rather than to focus on the commissioning of hospital care, continued with the formation of PCGs and then primary care trusts (PCTs) (Dowswell, Harrison and Wright, 2002, Lewis, 2004).

On the face of it one could conclude that the GPs in this case study were keen to take on the duties of corporate rationalizers, which are to challenge how health care is currently produced and distributed. The introduction of the GP fundholding scheme allowed GPs to engage in the activities of corporate rationalization but that is not to say that the GPs seized this opportunity; one must differentiate between the potentials that a structural change such as the GP fund-holding scheme provides and what actually occurs on the ground. The reasons why the GPs may not have utilized the tools within the GP fundholding scheme to engage in the process of corporate rationalization will be discussed further.

First, there are the differences in the levels of enthusiasm toward the fundholding scheme among the multifund GPs. The multifund contained a majority of uninterested GPs who viewed joining the fundholding scheme as inevitable and saw the multifund structure as a way of joining the scheme without having to be overly involved in the mechanics of fundholding. Chapter 5 illustrated the fact that the majority of the multifund GPs were uninvolved in a process which they viewed as largely managerial in nature. These unenthusiastic GPs were unlikely eagerly to pursue the mechanisms offered to them by the fundholding scheme in order to challenge the way hospital services were delivered. However, the data illustrated how some of the multifund GPs were interested in the opportunities to influence hospital services that they saw the fundholding scheme giving them. This was particularly true of the medical manager who had invested a considerable amount of time and effort into setting up the multi-fund. The findings of the first case study showed that a small core group of GPs had assumed responsibility for running the multifund, while the majority of the others had little or no involvement in the processes. This suggests that GPs who wanted to engage in the processes of corporate rationalization were given this opportunity by the fundholding scheme; however, the data from the first case study suggest that these types of GPs were in the minority. These findings agree with other studies into GP-led commissioning that have reported similar conclusions (Smith and Barnes, 2000).

Just as the medical profession as a whole is heterogeneous, so GPs differ; and this was also true of the multifund GPs. The heterogeneity of GPs was evident in the findings of research into the Total Purchasing Pilots (TPP) (Robinson, 1998). This was an experiment carried out towards the end of the 1992 Conservative administration which extended the fundholding scheme by giving participating practices the opportunity to contract for a wider range of health services than was available to conventional fundholders (Mays, Goodwin, Bevan and Wyke, 1997). This study reported that although the majority of participating GPs regarded the contracting process as important, there was a range of different reasons given for this. Some GPs felt that the contracting process gave them a greater opportunity to communicate with hospital consultants in order to gain their support for changes in hospital services. Other GPs felt the contracting process allowed them to negotiate from a position of strength and gave them the ability to shift contracts if their present providers were seen as intransigent. The evidence from this study would suggest that although the contracting process was perceived as offering fundholding GPs the opportunities to influence hospital consultants, the method of influence varied from practice to practice. Collaborative relationships between fundholding GPs and hospital consultants were as likely to result as combative ones. The evidence from the first case study suggested that while many GPs were eager to influence hospital services in theory, most of them were unwilling actively to exploit the opportunities offered to them by the fundholding scheme. However, there was a small minority that viewed the scheme as a welcome opportunity to address the perceived problems they saw in the hospital sector. This general lack of enthusiasm among most of the multifund GPs blunted the potential for the multifund to influence their local hospital services significantly.

The second factor that mitigated against the regulatory effects of the fundholding scheme and tended to lead to collaboration rather than confrontation between the multifund and the trust was the multifund's stated aim of supporting their local hospital. Another study reported informants giving similar reasons for participating in a total purchasing pilot consortium (Hurst, Harrison and Ride, 2000). This aim limited the multifund's desire to use the internal market and the contracting process either to move or threaten to move contracts to alternative providers in order to gain improvements from their local hospital trust. This meant that the already limited opportunities for competition, due to the lack of local alternative providers, were further blunted by the fact that the multifund did not want seriously to destabilize its local trust by withdrawing contracts. This factor was a significant impediment for the multifund, as even relatively minor switches in health care provision from one provider to another can have unintended knock-on effects for other services which can result in serious implications for a trust as a whole. The large degree of interconnectedness of hospital services made it difficult for GPs to withdraw their patronage from one unsatisfactory service without affecting other services they were keen to support. This mixture of structural and cultural factors constrained the multifund's ability significantly to influence hospital services and the GPs' abilities and desires to act as corporate rationalizers and challenge the dominant structural interests of the hospital consultants. This illustrates how a policy such as the fundholding scheme, which offers GPs the opportunity to influence many aspects of hospital services they were unhappy with, may not function as anticipated at the micro level where the policy is mediated within a complex cultural and structural context. These results illustrate the multi-layered quality of hospital consultants' dominance within the health care system which enables them to dilute the potential challenges that structural changes may contain.

However, this is not to say that the fundholding scheme did not bring about any changes within the hospital sector. Although many of the consultants felt that contracting in general and the quality standards in particular had had a very limited impact upon how they worked, there was evidence that pointed to the fact that the GPs had managed to make some gains. The data from the first case study in Chapter 4 provided evidence that some changes did occur in certain areas, which concurs with other empirical evidence about the impact of GP fundholders (Harrison and Choudhry, 1996). Both GPs and consultants stated that there had been reduced waiting times in the specialties of ophthalmology and ear, nose and throat. The speed and content of discharge summaries had improved and there had been an increase in the number of outreach clinics that were taking place in GP surgeries. There was also evidence of improvements on less concrete issues such as improved communication between GPs and hospital consultants. The evidence from both case studies would seem to suggest that fundholding GPs were able to challenge some practices of hospital consultants with which they were unhappy, however limited they were.

The above discussion illustrates that although certain changes were exacted from the trust, the multifund decided in both conscious and unconscious ways not to over-exploit the regulatory opportunities offered to it by the fundholding scheme. The prevailing dominance of the hospital consultants is further illustrated by the data in relation to the multifund's quality standards contained in Chapter 5. As far as these were concerned the hospital consultants displayed the medical profession's tactic of blocking unwelcome or threatening initiatives. This tactic is part of the medical profession's micro power, which has been described as

> ... *essentially conservative – it is a power to resist change that comes from outside, to resist not necessarily by battles at meetings and other 'first face' campaigns . . . but rather by silent, individualistic non-compliance – a 'second face' refusal to become engaged or involved.* (Harrison, Hunter, Marnoch and Pollitt, 1992, p. 140).

Many consultants stated that they had no knowledge of the quality standards, which agrees with other studies that have also reported on consultants' lack of involvement in contracting issues such as quality standards (Bensley, Bull and Haward, 1991). Consultants' lack of knowledge of the quality standards was probably a mixture of a lack of interest by them and poor communication of the standards within the trust. A study in the Yorkshire region reported that 32 per cent of consultants had had no discussions regarding quality standards, and only 29 per cent had discussed them in a formal and regular way. Of the consultants surveyed 63 per cent stated that their hospital had not organized even one event to discuss the hospital's contracting process (Bensley, Bull and Haward, 1991). The data from this study show how the hospital consultants largely ignored the multifund's quality standards or in some instances used them to their advantage in order to demand more resources to meet the standards. The hospital consultants' continued dominance would seem to lie more in the way that they have managed to prevent threats to them from emerging rather than having to defend themselves once threats had arisen. In Lukes' (1974) terms the hospital consultants at the micro level possess third dimensional power that enables them to determine *the perceptions, cognitions and preferences of others* (p. 24). The quality standards offer an example of this micro level power that the hospital consultants displayed.

The quality standards that the GPs contained within their outpatient contracts were mainly concerned with process-type issues rather than laying down clinical standards. Other studies have also reported on GPs' wishes to include quality specifications in contracts that address non-clinical issues such as the earlier arrival of discharge slips, the supply of medicines after discharge and the type of hospital doctor who should see new patients (Bowling, Jacobson, Southgate and Formby, 1991). The multifund GPs were on the whole reluctant to introduce clinically based standards into their contracts as they felt that this was a sensitive area where partnership rather than confrontation was the best way forward. This fact was reflected in the survey of health professionals that found that less than half of the GP respondents felt that the quality standards should cover clinical issues (Graph 5.3). Other studies into the content of quality specifications in health authorities' contracts also found that the specifications were generally broad in nature, did not specify any monitoring arrangements and contained no sanctions for the non-delivery of quality specifications (Gray and Donaldson, 1996).

However, there was evidence from both case studies that although the hospital consultants' dominance is still present, a more equitable relationship had developed between the two branches of medicine. This would seem to suggest that general practice as a specialty was keen to re-establish itself within the medical hierarchy, a tendency that Alford (1975) argued could occur, stating that

> . . . the potential specialties which are out in the professional cold, or losing ground, are forced in their own self-interest to fight back, regardless of the possible cost to the legitimacy of a professional united front . . . (p. 198)

It is difficult to determine whether this situation has been the result of GPs gaining power or hospital consultants suffering a decline. Perhaps the situation is more complex and power in these circumstances is not a 'zero sum', that is to say the GPs' gain may not have occurred at the expense of the consultants. For example, the fact that

the multifund GPs had managed to speed up their receipt of discharge summaries from consultants does not necessarily imply that
this requirement affects the consultants' power. The quicker dis-
patching of discharge summaries may have resulted from the fact
that the consultants had been supplied with greater secretarial input,
rather than requiring them to work more rapidly or differently in
response to the GPs' demands. Viewing the GP–hospital consultant
relationship as one of 'give and take' is perhaps an over simplistic
approach to what is in practice a more complex situation.

Another important result from both case studies was that the level
of communication between GPs and consultants had increased considerably and both sides felt they had a better level of understanding
of each other's situation. This rise in communication may help bring
GPs and hospital consultants together into a more united medical
group in order to gain improvements in both of their situations
rather than prompting GPs to challenge their medical colleagues
who work in the hospital sector. This result is perhaps a sign of the
hospital profession as a whole uniting as professional monopolizers
in order both to resist unwelcome challenges and extract concessions
from the traditional agents of corporate rationalization, that is,
management. This is a process that Alford detected when he argued
that

> *In particular historical periods, these conflicts among specialty
> groups or between specialists and the general practitioners may be
> the most visible and important ones, but this does not contradict
> the general interest which all segments of the professional mon-
> opolists share in maintaining an institutional framework which
> guarantees the continuation of the **principle** of professional
> autonomy and control, regardless of internal conflict over the dis-
> tribution of the powers and privileges.* (p. 197, emphasis in the
> original)

The data on health care quality in Chapter 5 illustrated some
important differences between GPs and consultants, indicating how
the two branches of medicine differ on the complex issue of health
care quality. GPs were mainly concerned with process-type issues
such as waiting times for outpatient appointments and the convenience of services in the form of outreach clinics. Hospital consultants,
on the other hand, were more concerned with the effectiveness of
treatment in terms of outcomes. These differing views were also evident in the health professionals' survey results of the first case study
and similar results have been reported in other studies (Whynes and

Reed, 1994). These results suggest that GPs accurately reflect their patients' priorities, a feature that was again borne out in the two surveys, which showed that patients' concerns over waiting times found resonance with GPs who also raised this as an important quality issue. These differences may be a reflection of the fact that hospital consultants have a greater degree of detachment from their patients who are professionally referred to them and who are ultimately referred back to the care of the GP. GPs, on the other hand, see self-referred patients and when referring them on to a consultant they act as their advocate and resume their care upon discharge. The data illustrate how GPs as the more dominant structural interest group are advocating the interests of the repressed community.

It was noted in Chapter 2 how the GP fundholding scheme provided GPs with the vehicle upon which to challenge the way hospital services were provided and attempt to orientate them more towards their patients' priorities. It was detailed in Chapter 2 that the Conservative government's GP fundholding scheme saw the GP as a suitable proxy for patients. The government felt that the fundholding scheme would strengthen GPs' influence over hospital services in general and consultants in particular. One of the fundholding scheme's aims was to make the GP a more important player within the health care system. The data suggest that the GPs' concerns do more accurately reflect those of their patients. Furthermore, there was evidence that the GPs as part of fundholding practices were able in some instances successfully to reconfigure services in order that they could be more convenient for patients. The issue of outreach clinics in GP surgeries was a good example of this. Although many of the hospital consultants did not consider outreach clinics to represent a good quality service, they were forced to provide them to GPs who, in the main, regarded them as offering a more effective and convenient service for their patients. This illustrates how the views of hospital consultants were successfully challenged by GPs who used patients' wishes in order to modify consultants' behaviour, even when the research evidence on outreach clinics tended to support the consultants' negative view of them (Bailey, Black and Wilkin, 1994; Hurst, Harrison and Ride, 2000). The case of outreach clinics is significant because it illustrates how GPs were able to use the contracting process to force hospital consultants to do an activity that they did not consider important.

Although discharge summaries and outreach clinics were two examples where fundholding GPs were able successfully to challenge the way hospital consultants worked, these seem to be somewhat

isolated incidents. These instances may represent the limited concessions that hospital consultants were prepared to make to GPs in
order to maintain their dominance within the health care system as a
whole. Furthermore, the data from both the semi-structured interviews and the health professionals' survey in the first case study
clearly show that there were various intraprofessional differences
between GPs and hospital consultants on a number of issues. However, the data suggest, particularly from the second case study, that as
time went by the relationship between the GP fundholders and their
local providers matured, and developed into an atmosphere of co-
operation rather than of confrontation. This is perhaps a reflection
of the GPs becoming increasingly aware of the limits of the fundholding scheme and recognizing that their influence over hospital
services and consultants was limited. It may also be a recognition on
the part of GPs that their long-term interests are better served by
being part of the professional monopoly than by attempting to
challenge it as corporate rationalizers.

The first case study suggests that some GPs were initially willing to
use the mechanisms that the fundholding scheme offered them in
order to make changes to some of the hospital practices with which
they were dissatisfied. The data illustrated instances where some GPs
were acting as corporate rationalizers and challenging the hospital
consultants. The data also illustrate that they were successful in certain areas, and that in general GPs managed to gain a more equitable
relationship with hospital consultants than was evident before the
1991 reforms, even though this was not obviously at the expense of
the consultants. With the passage of time the GP informants realized
that their influence over hospital services was limited through the
internal market and that any long-term changes were best achieved
by co-operating with their hospital colleagues rather than confronting them. The second case study provided the opportunity of
investigating whether the changes to the intraprofessional relations
that had appeared during the fundholding scheme were transient or
would have a more enduring quality.

THE LEGACY OF FUNDHOLDING

The second case study sought to examine whether the changes that
had been identified via the multifund case study were intrinsically
associated with the fundholding scheme or whether they were of a
more long-term nature and thus somewhat independent from or

resistant to the structural changes that then occured under the new Labour administration, such as the dissolution of GP fundholding and ending of the internal market. Mays *et al.* (1997) who examined the extension of the GP fundholding scheme into total purchasing pilots suggested that primary care-based purchasing could only be effective if it had some 'bite' in the form of contestability and financial leverage, which some argue was not initially evident within the new primary care structures set up by the Labour government (Robinson, 1998). However, this situation may change with the introduction of recent initiatives such as payment by results and patient choice (Department of Health, 2002b; Department of Health, 2003a)

The second chapter suggested that the 1999 Labour-inspired NHS reforms – and certainly those developed during Blair's second term – were in many respects a continuation of those ushered in by the Conservative government in 1991. For example, by continuing to involve GPs in commissioning health services, the new administration accepted that this had been a positive development. The second case study, which was conducted in the first half of the year 2000, two years after the fundholding scheme had been abolished and one year into the existence of PCGs, sought to examine this proposition. The timing of the data-gathering meant that the informants were able to reflect on their experiences of the fundholding scheme and their initial perceptions of the new primary care structures could also be examined.

Chapter 4 indicated that the informants' perceptions of the fundholding scheme in the second case study were similar to those uncovered in the first case study, but there were also some important differences in emphasis. The second case study informants did not report a high level of confrontation between primary and secondary care organizations and particularly between fundholding GPs and hospital consultants. This perception of good relations between primary and secondary care during the fundholding period has been reported by other studies (Hurst, Harrison and Ride, 2000). These findings add weight to the trend that was identified in the second round of interviews of the first case study, namely, that after an initial period of confrontation between GP purchasers and providers, relationships had increasingly become typified by collaboration and partnership as the constraints faced by both providers and purchasers were increasingly recognized by all parties involved in the contracting process.

The data relating to the experiences of fundholding from the second case study further illustrated that these GPs had also managed to make some changes to the hospital services. There were clear examples given by all the informants (including the consultants themselves) of the consultants having to be more responsive to GPs, and both the GPs and the hospital consultants saw this as a change to what had occurred before the introduction of the fundholding scheme. This increased level of interaction between the two sections of the medical profession had led to a greater understanding of each other's work and an appreciation of one another's pressures. The nature of GP–hospital consultant communication had altered under the fundholding scheme: the interactions were no longer purely clinical but were increasingly concerned with issues relating to service organization. These findings are in agreement with the evidence gained in the second-round interviews of the first case study and have been reported in other GP fundholding studies (Hurst, Harrison and Ride, 2000; Lewis, 1998). The importance of the contracting process and fundholding GPs' ability to shift contracts due to the fact that they could control their practice budget was also illustrated in the second case study. Many of the initiatives such as the marketing strategy and improvements in service accessibility that the hospital trust had embarked upon were in response to contract threats from the fundholding GPs. This is an indication that if these threats are no longer present GPs may find it more difficult to influence the providers. This situation may have prompted the Labour administration into implementing the new policy initiatives in the areas of GP commissioning, patient choice and payment by results, which might provide the necessary leverage.

Data from the second case study confirmed other commentators' views that the fundholding system had created what had been termed a 'two-tier' health service where patients who were registered with fundholding practices received speedier hospital treatment than those registered with non-fundholding practices (Goodwin, 1998). Both non-fundholding and fundholding GP informants confirmed this aspect of the scheme. This evidence also suggests that the advantages that fundholding GPs were obtaining for their patients were associated with their fundholding status and would thus disappear once fundholding was abolished. Indeed, this inequity between fundholding and non-fundholding practices was cited as a reason for the Labour government's desire for a universal primary care structure as opposed to the previously voluntary GP fundholding scheme (Department of Health, 1997). It remains to be seen whether these inequities reappear with New Labour's introduction of indicative budgets for GPs in 2005. However, there was a counter-view to this from the data which suggested that although patients registered with fundholding practices gained the most, other patients registered with non-GP fundholders also benefited as hospitals raised their level of service for all patients regardless of the fundholding status of their GP. The fundholding informants stated that they had not only been able to improve hospital services for their patients but they had also improved the services their patients could receive in the GP practice, a point that was also illustrated in the first case study by the extension of outreach clinics into GP surgeries.

An important point made by the managers who were interviewed in the second case study was that many of the positive changes that fundholding GPs had managed to make to hospital services were associated with the fact that they were 'marginal purchasers'. That is to say, they were only responsible for purchasing 20 per cent of services and this fact allowed them to be more flexible and use the contracting system to gain better services for their patients. These managers felt that such advantages might be lost within the new PCG and PCT structures that would be responsible for purchasing all of their population's health care and as a consequence may be less flexible in their commissioning of health services.

In summary, the informants' reflections upon the fundholding scheme in the second case study confirmed many of the findings that emerged from the multifund study and provided evidence on aspects such as a two-tier health system that had perhaps not emerged in the earlier multifund study. The second case study also provided evidence that suggested that many of the advantages that fundholding GPs had obtained were intrinsically linked to their fundholding status and could thus disappear as GP fundholding vanished. So what did the second case study tell us about the future and the possible impacts of the new primary care organizations?

Most GPs who had been part of the fundholding scheme felt that although its abolition was necessary because of the resulting inequities, its demise would mean that their influence and freedom would be reduced; similar perceptions by some GPs have been reported in other studies of PCGs (Dowswell, Harrison and Wright, 2002). Interestingly, the hospital consultants' perceptions were that the creation of PCGs and PCTs would further enhance the influence of GPs due to the fact that they will be in charge of commissioning all their population's health services rather than a marginal 20 per cent as was the case under the fundholding scheme. This contrasts with the views of the health care managers who felt that it was the very fact that GP fundholders were marginal purchasers that gave them the influence they had within the previous arrangements. It may be that the new primary care structures where a group of GP practices come together will be more effective in influencing a local trust by representing a greater critical mass of GPs rather than a single GP fundholding practice. The potential for the new primary care structures to have a greater influence within the NHS is certainly there at least in terms of resources, as PCTs now control 75 per cent of the NHS budget (Ham, 2004). However, these new structures will only be able to do this if they manage to achieve a level of internal coherence that will enable them to act as an effective group rather than a loosely associated collection of GP practices, as was the situation in the multifund case study. Greater cohesion may develop, as indicated by a case study of the development of clinical governance within a PCG which reported that the PCG structure had helped promote a greater degree of collaboration between practices (Baeza and Campbell, 2001; Baeza, 2004). There was also a view from the consultants in the second case study that conflicts of interest might occur in the new primary care structures due to the fact that they will be responsible for both purchasing and providing health services.

Both GPs and consultants agreed that the likely outcome of this would be that more health care would be provided in primary care settings. If this trend develops in practice it may be a sign of a changing power base from the hospital towards the GP surgery. Rather than gaining their influence from attempting to control the secondary care sector and thus act as a new corporate rationalizer, GPs may in the future attain more power by directly controlling services that are provided within their sphere of influence, which is primary care. This could be a signal that GPs in the new primary care organizations will be reverting back to their professional monopolizer past as they seek to become dominant within these new increasingly influential primary care structures. However, the hospital's status as the power base within the British health care system means that if this transfer of power happens at all it will occur only slowly.

The trend of bringing more health care into primary care settings was greatly accelerated by fundholding GPs who used their budgets either to employ staff such as counsellors directly or to purchase certain diagnostic services that would previously have been controlled by the hospital. The data from the second case study suggested that this trend is set to expand even further with the advent of PCGs and PCTs. This development is likely to have an impact on both the intraprofessional relations between GPs and hospital consultants and within the GP group itself. The implications for the GP–hospital consultant relationship is that a greater degree of trust will need to exist between these two groups to enable hospital consultants to delegate a greater extent of patient care to their GP colleagues. It may be that the new equality between GPs and hospital consultants that developed under the fundholding scheme will continue and new mechanisms such as shared protocols and guidelines may be used, enabling a greater amount of health care to be undertaken in the GP practice or other primary care settings. However, other studies have reported a significant degree of disagreement between hospital consultants and GPs on a number of important issues relating to the appropriate primary/secondary care divide. Marshall (1999) found disagreement between the two groups upon the degree of open access GPs should have to special investigations and to the extent that chronic diseases can be better managed by GPs in primary care settings than in specialist outpatient clinics. On the positive side, this same study also reported that GPs and hospital consultants agreed upon the fact that an equal ability was necessary to become a specialist or a GP and there was an acceptance by the hospital consultants that GPs should be able to influence the service provided by hospital specialists. These findings suggest that a better understanding is developing between GPs and hospital consultants but important disagreements as to the appropriate primary/secondary health care balance still exist.

The increase of work carried out in the primary care sector is also likely to have an impact upon GPs themselves. The second case study found examples of referrals occurring among GPs of the same PCG and there was a suggestion that this trend may increase in the future. By 2003 there were 1,250 GPs with special interests who were taking referrals from fellow GPs. These developments may create divisions within the GP population similar to those seen between GPs and hospital consultants in the past (Mahmood, 2001). An elite cadre of GPs may develop, thereby creating a more stratified GP population. It is likely that these elite GPs, and perhaps the medical profession more generally, will gain their status both from their clinical expertise and their managerial skills (Harrison and Ahmad, 2000). Again this trend may signify that clinicians are increasingly deriving prestige and power from their managerial prowess as well as from their clinical abilities, perhaps illustrating their growing need to display corporate rationalizer-type characteristics. These developments were illustrated in the data from the second case study where the GP

informants who were not involved in the PCG management com-
plained that they were not being kept informed of what was going on
and felt more constrained within the PCG structure than under the
fundholding scheme. On the other hand, the GP informants who
were members of the PCG board stated that GPs would have to
realize that they are no longer lone practitioners but that their
actions have implications for the wider GP group and their practice
would thus have to reflect this. These developments suggest that
GPs will become increasingly more managed, but the nature of this
management seems set to change. GPs who opt to become involved
in the management of the new primary care structures will be
increasingly responsible for managing the activities of their GP
colleagues, which will include the management of sensitive areas
such as poor performance and prescribing.

Mark (1991) has commented that although the medical profession
as a whole may question the degree to which it should become
involved in management, individual doctors may welcome greater
managerial responsibilities because of the potential benefits it could
afford them on a personal level. The new primary care structures
could make the practice of those GPs who are not managerially
engaged in PCTs to be increasingly determined by their GP colleagues who do choose to become involved in PCT management. At
the micro level this could imply that certain GPs will be adopting the
role of corporate rationalizers, both internally towards their GP colleagues and externally in relation to hospital consultants. The indica-
tions from other studies are that these developments were occurring
internally within PCGs, as individual GPs began to adopt managerial positions within these organizations (Baeza and Campbell, 2001;
Baeza, 2004). Policies such as clinical governance may contribute to
this trend as a central aim of this initiative is to make groups of
professionals accountable for each other's performance, replacing
individual responsibility for the quality of practice with a collective
one (Allen, 2000). There have, however, always been differences
within general practice, which were highlighted during the GP fundholding period when some GPs actively welcomed the initiative while
others shunned the scheme and set up alternative structures.

The new developments within primary care have created an
environment of ever greater divisions within general practice where
power is unevenly spread throughout the GP population (Lewis,
1998; Mahmood, 2001). If there is an increase in the establishment
of primary care-based services, as this study and others have suggested (Smith and Barnes, 2000), then the distribution of power and

influence among GPs will become increasingly important. However, this tendency could radically change as GPs' influence on management boards is now more diluted as a consequence of the broader professional composition of PCTs. Alongside these developments that may have accentuated the divisions within primary care there is also contrasting research evidence reporting that the new primary care organizations have increased the level of collaboration among GPs (Baeza and Campbell, 2001; Baeza, 2004; Smith, Regen, Shapiro and Baines, 2000; Smith and Barnes, 2000).

ALFORD REVISITED

Alford (1975) developed his theory of structural interests, which was examined in detail in Chapter 3, in order to explain the reform process in the New York City health system and it has been applied by others to study various changes in the NHS (Ham, 1981; Allsop, 1984; North 1998; North and Peckham, 2001). The dominant structural interests are those maintained by the existing structures and Alford identified the medical profession as representing the professional monopolizers who are the dominant structural interest within the health system. The corporate rationalizers who are represented by health service managers and government planners occupy the challenging structural interests. The final category in Alford's framework is that of repressed structural interests, which in the USA is represented by the section of the population who are either uninsured or without health care coverage. This structural interest does not transfer directly to the UK case where the NHS provides universal coverage to its population.

Chapter 1 illustrated how the history of the medical profession in the past hundred years has been typified by the division in British medicine between GPs and hospital consultants, resulting in the latter occupying the dominant structural interest *within* the medical profession. It was argued that the 1991 structural reforms of the NHS helped to accentuate the already significant divide and potentially change the intraprofessional relations between the two branches of medicine. The reforms provided the opportunity for GPs to become fundholders and as such challenge the dominance of hospital consultants. This study used Alford's framework in order to examine whether the NHS reforms of 1991 and 1999 led to structural realignments where GPs, firstly as GP fundholders and latterly within PCGs, became corporate rationalizers within the English NHS.

The data from this study have provided various examples where the GPs have shown certain corporate rationalizer-type characteristics by successfully challenging the work of hospital consultants and attempting to restrict their power, and there are also examples of hospital consultants defending their interests with the professional monopolizer's weaponry. However, at the same time, the GP fundholders were reluctant to use all their potential powers to challenge the work of hospital consultants. This reluctance seemed to be the result both of constraints within the GP group itself and of the hospital consultants' subtle use of the existing structures to legitimize their position. There was evidence from both case studies that the relationship between GPs and hospital consultants had become more evenly balanced. The evidence would suggest that the previous Conservative government's aim of strengthening GPs' influence within the health care system in general and hospital services in particular was achieved by the GP fundholding scheme. Furthermore, the data support the view that GPs were able to act as advocates for the repressed interests of the community as they shared common concerns that could be conveyed more powerfully within the fundholding scheme. However, both case studies illustrated how the quantity and quality of communication between GPs and hospital consultants had improved. There was evidence that the communication between GPs and hospital consultants had broadened from clinical discussions to issues relating to health service organization. These changes, coupled with a more equitable relationship, could result in a more united medical profession, which is better able to maintain its dominance within the NHS. This is to say that the GP fundholding scheme led to a degree of redistribution of power among the medical profession, which was then followed by a reunification of the two branches of medicine in order to maintain and defend their shared interests of professional autonomy and control (Alford, 1975, p.197). At this level of analysis Alford's framework is an instructive way to study the impact of the 1991 health care reforms by examining their influence in structural interest terms.

To what extent have the structural interests been reconfigured and to what extent can the results from this study be viewed as merely temporary readjustments within the dominant structural interests of the professional monopolizers? The second case study suggested that much of the increased influence of GPs was intrinsically linked to their fundholding status and could disappear with the scheme's demise. However, the fact that PCTs are now responsible for over 75 per cent of the health care budget and that an increasing number of procedures are being provided within primary care, may allow at least some GPs (particularly those who choose directly to commission services) to maintain and perhaps even increase their influence within the NHS. Some commentators have suggested that a process of professional restratification may occur within the GP population that could make predicting outcomes far more difficult (Mahmood, 2001).

By using Alford's structural interests approach one is able both to assess the extent to which GPs can be usefully seen as corporate rationalizers and to analyse how this will affect the intraprofessional relations of GPs and hospital consultants. However, it is perhaps when one wishes to look inside a primary care organization that Alford's framework becomes less instructive as it fails to illuminate the more subtle differences between stakeholders at this level, where allegiances may sway depending on the issue being considered (North and Peckham, 2001). It is perhaps here that it is more enlightening to examine these dynamics from Freidson's viewpoint of a stratified medical profession (Freidson, 1994, p.9).

A more stratified medical profession, where divisions occur both horizontally between secondary and primary care as well as vertically within these two sectors, may signal a weakened medical profession in general. However, on a micro level the situation is likely to be more complicated with individual winners and losers among the two branches of the profession itself. The scenario of a weakened medical profession in general was beginning to be illustrated in the second case study where the consultants, particularly, perceived that they were now subjected to a greater level of regulation. They felt these pressures coming from all sides: patients, managers and government. They saw the new quality agenda as having a regulatory edge to it and they also felt that the consumer voice was becoming stronger and more powerful. These may well just be the recognizable complaints from a still powerful profession that is positioning itself to block these emergent threats or a recognition on their part that their dominant position within the NHS is coming to an end. It will be important for future research to continue to investigate the intraprofessional relations both *between* GPs and hospital consultants and *within* these two sections of the medical profession since these two groups will continue to play significant roles in the development of the British health care system.

APPENDIX: METHODOLOGY

This study focused on the key actors' experiences and perceptions; hence a qualitative approach was adopted. A semi-structured interview schedule was developed for use in tape-recorded face-to-face interviews. The contracting process was used as the central theme in the first case study interviews to explore the informants' perceptions of the structural changes. The informants selected for interview were mainly those who were believed to have a direct or indirect impact on the contracting process. Figure A below presents a framework for the structure of the contracting process that was based on accounts derived from government policy documents (Department of Health, 1989a). It shows who and at what points the various actors might be involved in the contracting process.

The research reported in this book consisted of two case studies. The first case study was of a GP multifund in the south-east of England. The GPs were selected for interview by using a list that was supplied by the multifund. As well as providing the names and addresses of GPs this list contained various details of the practices, such as the number of partners and whether the GPs were registered as trainers or not. The purposive sample included GPs who reflected the full range of practices that formed the multifund so that the interviews could access the full range of GP perspectives. The GP sample therefore included GPs from both small and large practices, deprived and non-deprived areas, female and male doctors, urban and rural and training and non-training practices. The sample also included one fundholding GP who was outside the multifund structure and one non-fundholding GP. The hospital consultant informants were selected from lists supplied by the two main hospital trusts that the multifund purchased services from. They included physicians,

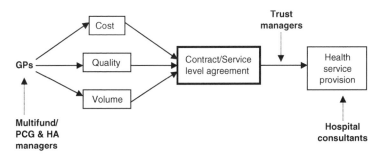

Figure A The contracting process

surgeons, senior consultants (for example medical directors and clinical directors) and less senior consultants. Including the contract and
outpatient managers from the multifund's two main trusts as well as
managers from the host health authority and the multifund's central
office completed the sample in this case study as shown in Table A
below. This first case study consisted of two rounds of interviews
that were carried out between December 1995 and May 1996 and
between March and June 1997 respectively.

In the second smaller case study, the data-gathering took place
between March and May 2000 and focused upon a primary care
group (PCG) in the south-east of England. Figure A above illustrates the main stakeholders that were identified in the first case study;
although some of the labels had changed, the types of informants
remained the same. The purposive sample of the second case study

Table A First case study informants

OCCUPATION	*1st ROUND*	*2nd ROUND*
Multifund GPs	7	5
Non-multifund GPFH	1	1
Non GPFH	1	1
Multifund managers	2	1
Other multifund manager	1	0
Hospital consultants	6	5
Hospital contract managers	2	2
Outpatients managers	2	2
Health authority manager	1	1
FHSA manager	1	0
TOTALS	**24**	**18**

was devised so that it included a similar range of informants as in the first case study. The final sample consisted of a range of PCG GPs from small and large practices, those set in more and less deprived areas and included PCG board members as well as those that can be regarded as 'rank and file' GPs (5); a range of hospital consultants from different specialties and different levels of seniority from the PCG's main provider trust (5); and senior managers from the PCG, the main provider trust and the host health authority (3). The broad aim of this case study was to examine the GP–hospital consultant relationship following the demise of the GP fundholding scheme and the introduction of PCGs. This case study sought to study whether the 1999 health care reforms would simply build upon those of 1991 or would herald a new phase in the intra-professional relations within the medical profession. The interviews in the second case study examined the informants' perspectives of the 1999 primary care reforms and how they compared and contrasted with those of 1991. This second case study provided empirical evidence of the impact of the abolition of the internal market and the GP fundholding scheme upon the primary–secondary care interface.

The transcripts from both case studies were analysed through multiple readings of the data. The data were initially read so as to become familiar with the material and then to identify emergent themes inductively. The data were then rearranged into common areas. In this thematic form the data were re-read so as to construct a sequential argument which is illustrated by selected quotations (Harvey, 1990). The qualitative methods computer programme *Atlas ti* (Muhr, 1997) was used to aid this process.

THE SURVEYS

The quantitative element of the study consisted of a survey of a random sample of recent users of the outpatient services and a second survey of the total population of health care professionals involved directly or indirectly in the provision of outpatient services. The patient postal questionnaire investigated outpatient users' awareness, their views of the acceptability and importance of the quality standards used by the multifund in its outpatient contract, as well as the levels of satisfaction with their experience of their last outpatient visit. A systematic sample of 610 patients was extracted from the patient lists of the multifund GP practices. The multifund was able to provide a list of patients over the age of 18 years from all its GP practices who had attended an outpatient appointment at the multifund's main provider trust in the past four months. Every tenth patient from this list was selected and their patient record was identified so as to obtain their postal address. After sending out two reminders and a new questionnaire the user survey concluded with an achieved sample of 354, which represented a 58 per cent response rate.

The outpatient manager of the multifund's main provider trust provided the names of all the professionals who were either directly or indirectly involved in providing outpatient services. This method identified a sample of 213 professionals, which included all the consultants who had outpatient clinics, the outpatient nurses and the hospital managers who had any links with the outpatient services. As far as the purchasing side was concerned, all the multifund GPs, practice nurses and fundholding managers were included in the survey. The questionnaire that was mailed to the health professionals focused on their awareness and the acceptability and importance of the quality standards adopted by the multifund in the contract for outpatient services. After sending out two reminders and a new questionnaire to non-responders the achieved sample was 127, representing an overall response rate of 60 per cent. Table B below illustrates the breakdown of the response rates for the health care professionals.

Table B shows a disappointing response rate from GPs, a common feature of GP surveys which can be attributed to the high number of questionnaires they receive. It indicates that conclusions from the survey for this group must be treated with a degree of caution. However, the fact that at least one GP from 14 of the 16 practices within

Table B   Health care professionals' response rate

OCCUPATION	*NUMBER SENT*	*COMPLETED RETURNS*	*RESPONSE RATE (%)*
Consultant	71	44	62
Hospital Nurse	3	3	100
Hospital Manager	16	11	69
GP	65	31	48
Practice Nurse	40	27	68
Fundholding manager	18	11	61
TOTALS	**213**	**127**	**60**

the multifund responded to the questionnaire insured that there was a good representation from the range of the multifund's practices.

SUMMARY

This study utilized both qualitative and quantitative methods within a case study designed to investigate how the health policies implemented in the 1990s affected the intraprofessional relationships of GPs and hospital consultants in the English NHS. This research consisted of two phases: the first phase involved a case study of a GP fundholding multifund and the second phase was a case study of a PCG. The first case study examined the impact of a set of quality standards that were contained within the outpatient contracts that were negotiated between the GP multifund and its main hospital trust providers. This case study consisted of two rounds of semi-structured interviews with a purposive sample of informants, non-participant observation of contract meetings and two questionnaire surveys of health care professionals and patients. The second phase of the study involved a case study of a PCG in order to assess the early effects of the Labour government's health policy agenda upon the relationship of GPs and hospital consultants.

REFERENCES

Abbott, S., Harrison, S. and Walsh, N. (1999) Total purchasing in primary care: three case studies, *Journal of Management in Medicine*, **13**: 365–72.

Alford, R. (1975) *Health Care Politics*. Chicago: University of Chicago Press.

Allen, P. (2000) Accountability for clinical governance: developing collective responsibility for quality in primary care, *British Medical Journal*, **321**: 608–11.

Allsop, J. (1984) *Health Policy and the National Health Service*. London: Longman.

Allsop, J. (1995) *Health Policy and the NHS: Towards 2000*. London: Longman.

Appleby, J., Smith, P., Ranade, W., Little, V. and Robinson, R. (1994) Monitoring managed competition, in R. Robinson and J. Le Grand (eds) *Evaluating the NHS Reforms*. London: Kings Fund.

Audit Commission (1996) *What the Doctor Ordered: A Study of GP Fundholders in England and Wales*. London: HMSO.

Audit Commission (2000) *The PCG Agenda*. London: Audit Commission.

Baeza, J. I. (2004) Managing poor performance in a primary care group: the GP perspective, *British Journal of Health Care Management*, **10**: 78–81.

Baeza, J. and Calnan, M. (1999) Whose Quality? Different interest groups' perspectives on health care quality, in H. Davies, M. Malek, A. Neilson and M. Tavakoli (eds) *Managing Quality and Controlling Costs: Strategic Issues in Health Care Management*. Aldershot: Ashgate.

Baeza, J. and Campbell, J. (2001) *Developing Clinical Governance in a*

Primary Care Group. London: Department of General Practice and Primary Care, King's College.

Bailey, J., Black, M. and Wilkin, D. (1994) Specialised outreach clinics in general practice, *British Medical Journal*, 308: 1083–6.

Bensley, D., Bull, A. and Haward, R. (1991) Consultants' involvement in the contracting process in the Yorkshire region, *British Medical Journal*, 303: 95.

Best, G. (1983) Performance indicators: a precautionary tale for unit managers, in I. Wickings (ed.) *Effective Unit Management*. London: Kings Fund.

Bowling, A., Jacobson, B., Southgate, L. and Formby, J. (1991) General practitioners' views on quality specifications for outpatient referrals and care contracts, *British Medical Journal*, 303: 292–4.

British Medical Association (1965) Charter for the family doctor, *British Medical Journal*, 3138: 89.

Britten, N. (2000) Qualitative interviews in health care research, in *Qualitative Research in Health Care*, 2nd edn, ed. C. Pope and N. Mays. London: BMJ Books.

Brooks, T. and Pitt, C. (1990) The standard bearers, *The Health Service Journal*, 30 August.

Bryman, A. (1988) *Quantity and Quality in Social Research*. London: Unwin Hyman.

Butcher, T. (1995) *Delivering Welfare: The Governance of the Social Services in the 1990s*. Buckingham: Open University Press.

Butler, F. and Pirie, M. (1988) *The Health of Nations*. London: Adam Smith Institute.

Butler, J. (1993) Origins and early development, in R. Robinson and J. Le Grand (eds) *Evaluating the NHS Reforms*. Hermitage: Policy Journals.

Butler, J. and Calnan, M. (1987) *Too Many Patients?* Aldershot: Avebury.

Calnan, M. (1981) *Coping with accidents and emergencies, a study of how the community uses the hospital accident and emergency department*. Unpublished PhD Thesis. Templeman Library, University of Kent at Canterbury, UK.

Calnan, M. and Williams, S. (1995) Challenges to professional autonomy in the United Kingdom? The perceptions of general practitioners, *International Journal of Health Services*, 25: 219–41.

Carr-Saunders, A. M. and Wilson, D. A. (1933) *The Professions*. Oxford: The Clarendon Press.

Cartwright, A. and Anderson, R. (1979) *Patients and their Doctors 1977: Report on Some Changes in General Practice between 1964*

and 1977 for the Royal Commission on the National Health Service.
London: The Royal College of General Practitioners.

Cawson, A. (1982) *Corporatism and Welfare*. London: Heinemann.

Centre for the Evaluation of Public Policy and Practice (1992) *Considering Quality: An Analytical Guide to the Literature on Quality and Standards in the Public Services*. Brunel: Brunel University.

Chisholm, J. (1998) Primary care and the NHS white papers, *British Medical Journal*, **316**: 1687–8.

Cho, H-J. (2000) Traditional medicine, professional monopoly and structural interests: a Korean case, *Social Science and Medicine*, **50**: 123–35.

Clarke, J., Gewirtz, S. and McLaughlin, E. (2000) Reinventing the Welfare State, in J. Clarke, S. Gewirtz, and E. McLaughlin (eds) *New Managerialism, New Welfare?* London: Sage.

Cowton, C. and Drake, J. (1999) Went fundholding, going commissioning? Some evidence-based reflections on the prospects for primary care groups, *Public Management and Money*, April–June.

Dahl, R. (1961) *Who Governs?* Yale: Yale University Press.

Department of Health (1986) *Primary Health Care: An Agenda for Discussion*, Cmnd. 9771. London: HMSO.

Department of Health (1987) *Promoting Better Health*, Cm. 249. London: HMSO.

Department of Health (1989a) *General Practice in the NHS: The 1990 Contract*. London: HMSO.

Department of Health (1989b) *Practice Budgets for General Medical Practitioners*, Working for Patients, Working Paper 3. London: HMSO.

Department of Health (1989c) *NHS Consultants: Appointments, Contracts and Distinction Awards*, Working for Patients, Working Paper 7. London: HMSO.

Department of Health (1989d) *Medical Audit*, Working for Patients, Working Paper 6. London: HMSO.

Department of Health (1989e) *Resource Management Initiative*. London: HMSO.

Department of Health (1989f) *Funding and Contracts for Hospital Services*, Working for Patients, Working Paper 5. London: HMSO.

Department of Health (1989g) *Working for Patients*, Cm 555. London: HMSO.

Department of Health (1991) *The Patient's Charter*. London: HMSO.

Department of Health (1992) *The Health of the Nation, A Strategy for Health in England*, Cm 1986. London: HMSO.

Department of Health (1997) *The New NHS: Modern, Dependable*, Cm 3807. London: HMSO.

Department of Health (1998) *A First Class Service*. London: HMSO.

Department of Health (2000a) *The NHS Plan: A Plan for Investment, a Plan for Reform*. London: HMSO.

Department of Health (2000b) *National Service Framework for Coronary Heart Disease*. London: Department of Health.

Department of Health (2001a) *Assuring the Quality of Medical Practice*. London: Department of Health.

Department of Health (2001b) *Primary Care, General Practice and the NHS Plan*. London: Department of Health.

Department of Health (2001c) *Shifting the Balance of Power within the NHS*. London: Department of Health.

Department of Health (2002a) *A Guide to NHS Foundation Trusts*. London: Department of Health.

Department of Health (2002b) *Payment by Results*. London: Department of Health.

Department of Health (2003a) *Building on the Best: Choice, Responsiveness and Equity in the NHS*. London: Department of Health.

Department of Health (2003b) *Delivering Investment in General Practice*. London: Department of Health.

Department of Health (2004a) *Practice Based Commissioning. Engaging Practices in Commissioning*. London: Department of Health.

Department of Health (2004b) *The NHS Improvement Plan*. London: Department of Health.

Department of Health (2004c) *Consultant Contract*. London: Department of Health.

Derber C. (1982) The proletarianization of the professional, in C. Derber (ed.) *Professionals as Workers*. Boston: G. K. Hall.

Dingwall, R. and Fenn, P. (1992) Introduction, in R. Dingwall and P. Fenn (eds) *Quality and Regulation in Health Care: International Experiences*. London: Routledge.

Dixon, J. (1994) Can there be fair funding for fundholding practices?, *British Medical Journal*, **308**: 772–5.

Dixon, J., Dinwoodie, M., Hodson, D. *et al.* (1994) Distribution of NHS funds between fundholding and non-fundholding practices, *British Medical Journal*, **309**: 30–34.

Dixon, J. and Glennerster, H. (1995) What do we know about fundholding in general practice?, *British Medical Journal*, **314**: 216–19.

Dixon, J., Holland, P. and Mays, N. (1998) Primary care: core values. Developing primary care: Gatekeeping, commissioning and managed care. *British Medical Journal*, **317**: 125–8.

Dohler, M. (1989) Physicians' professional autonomy in the welfare state, in G. Freddi and J. Bjorkman (eds) *Controlling Medical Professionals*. London: Sage.

Donabedian, A. (1980) *Explorations in Quality Assessment and Monitoring. Volume 1: The Definition of Quality and Approaches to its Assessment*. Michigan: Health Administration Press.

Dowling, B. (1997) Effect of fundholding on waiting times: database study, *British Medical Journal*, **315**: 290–92.

Dowling, B., Wilkin, D and Smith, S (2003) Organizational development and governance of primary care, in B. Dowling and C. Glendinning (eds) *The New Primary Care*. Maidenhead: Open University Press.

Dowswell, G., Harrison, S. and Wright, J. (2002) The early days of primary care groups: General Practitioners' perceptions, *Health and Social Care in the Community*, **10**: 46–54.

Elston, M. A. (1991) The politics of professional power: medicine in a changing health service, in J. Gabe and M. Calnan (eds) *The sociology of the health service*. London: Routledge.

Enthoven, A. (1985) *Reflections on the Management of the NHS*, Occasional paper 5. London: Nuffield Provincial Hospitals Trust.

Exworthy, M. and Halford, S. (1999) Assesment and conclusions, in M. Exworthy and S. Halford (eds) *Professionals and the New Managerialism in the Public Sector*. Buckingham: Open University Press.

Ferlie, E. (1997) Large-scale organizational and managerial change in health care: a review of the literature, *Journal of Health Services Research and Policy*, **2**: 180–88.

Fielding, N. and Fielding, J. (1986) *Linking Data*. Beverly Hills: Sage.

Flynn, R. (1992) *Structures of Control in Health Management*. London: Routledge.

Flynn, R. and Williams, G. (1997a) Contracting for health, in R. Flynn and G. Williams (eds) *Contracting for Health*. Oxford: Oxford University Press.

Flynn, R. and Williams, G. (1997b) *Contracting for Health*. Oxford: Oxford University Press.

Flynn, R., Williams, G. and Pickard, S. (1996) *Markets and Networks: Contracting in Community Health Services*. Buckingham: Open University Press.

Forsyth G. (1973) *Doctors and State Medicine*. London: Pitman.

Freidson, E. (1970) *Profession of Medicine: a Study of the Sociology of Applied Knowledge*. New York: Dodd Mead.

Freidson, E. (1986) *Professional Powers*. Chicago: University of Chicago Press.

Freidson, E. (1994) *Professionalism Reborn*. Cambridge: Polity Press.

Fulop, N., Allen, P., Clarke, A. and Black, N. (2001) Issues in studying the organisation and delivery of health services, in N. Fulop, P. Allen, A. Clarke and N. Black (eds) *Studying the Organisation and Delivery of Health Services*. London: Routledge.

Gill, D. (1971) The British National Health Service: professional determinants of administrative structure, *International Journal of Health Services*, **1**: p. 342–53.

Glaser, B. and Strauss A. L. (1967) *The Discovery of Grounded Theory*. Chicago: Aldine.

Glendinning, C. (1999) GPs and contracts: bringing general practice into primary care, *Social Policy and Administration*, **33**: 115–31.

Glennerster, H., Matsaganis, M., Owens, P. and Hancock, S. (1993) Implementing GP fundholding: wild card or winning hand?, in R. Robinson and J. Le Grand (eds) *Evaluating the NHS Reforms*. London: Kings Fund.

Glennerster, H., Matsaganis, M., Owens, P. and Hancock, S. (1994) *Implementing GP Fundholding: wild card or winning hand?* Buckingham: Open University Press.

Goode, W. J. (1960) Encroachment, Charlatanism and the emerging profession: psychology, medicine and sociology, *American Sociological Review*, **XXV**: 902–14.

Goodwin, N. (1998) GP fundholding, in J. Le Grand, N. Mays and J-A. Mulligan (eds) *Learning from the NHS Internal Market*. London: King's Fund.

Gough, I. (1979) *The Political Economy of the Welfare State*. London: Macmillan.

Graffy, J. and Williams, J. (1994) Purchasing for all: an alternative to fundholding, *British Medical Journal*, **308**: 391–4.

Gray, D. (1979) *A System of Training for General Practice*. London: Royal College of General Practitioners.

Gray, D. (1992) History of the Royal College of General Practitioners – the first 40 years, *British Journal of General Practice*, **42**: 29–35.

Gray, D. and Donaldson, L. J. (1996) Improving the quality of health care through contracting: a study of health authority practice, *Quality in Health Care*, **5**: 201–5.

Great Britain, Parliament (2000) *Health Act*. London: Stationery Office.

Green, D. (1988) *Everyone a Private Patient*. London: Institute of Economic Affairs.

Griffiths, R. (1983) *The NHS Management Inquiry Report*. London: DHSS.

Grol, R. (1990) National standard setting for quality of care in general practice: attitudes of general practitioners and response to a set of standards, *British Journal of General Practice*, **40**: 361–4.

Grol, R. (1993) Development of guidelines for general practice care, *British Journal of General Practice*, **43**: 146–51.

Guardian (2001) Time for compromise: 24 February.

Ham, C. (1981) *Policy Making in the National Health Service*. Basingstoke: Macmillan.

Ham, C. (1985) *Health Policy in Britain*. Basingstoke: Macmillan.

Ham, C. (1996) Contestability: a middle path for health care, *British Medical Journal*, **312**: 70–71.

Ham, C. (1997) *Management and Competition in the NHS*. Abingdon: Radcliffe Medical Press.

Ham, C. (2004) *Health Policy in Britain*. Basingstoke: Macmillan.

Harrison, S. (1994) *National Health Service Management in the 1980s*. Aldershot: Avebury.

Harrison, S. (1999) Clinical autonomy and health policy: past and future, in M. Exworthy and S. Halford (eds) *Professionals and the New Managerialism in the Public Sector*. Buckingham: Open University Press.

Harrison, S. and Ahmad, W. (2000) Medical autonomy and the UK state, *Sociology*, **34**: 129–46.

Harrison, S. and Choudhry, N. (1996) General practice fundholding in the UK National Health Service: Evidence to date, *Journal of Public Health Policy*, **17**: 331–46.

Harrison, S., Hunter, D., Marnoch, G. and Pollitt, C. (1992) *Just Managing: Power and Culture in the National Health Service*. Basingstoke: Macmillan.

Harrison, S., Hunter, D. and Pollitt, C. (1990) *The Dynamics of British Health Policy*. London: Unwin.

Harrison S., Pohlman C, and Mercer G. (1994) Concept of clinical freedom amongst English physicians, EAPHSS Conference paper 8/6/94.

Harrison, S. and Pollitt, C. (1994) *Controlling Health Professionals*. Buckingham: Open University Press

Harvey, L. (1990) *Critical Social Research*. London: Unwin Hyman.

Haywood, S. and Alaszewski, A. (1980) *Crisis in the Health Service*. London: Croom Helm.

Hogarth-Scott, S. and Wright, G. (1997) Is quality of health care changing? GPs' views, *Journal of Management in Medicine*, **11**: 302–11.

Hoggett, P. (1991) A new management in the public sector?, *Policy and Politics*, **19**: 243–56.

Hollingsworth, J. (1986) *A Political Economy of Medicine: Great Britain and the United States*. Baltimore: The Johns Hopkins University Press.

Honigsbaum F. (1979) *The Division in British Medicine*. London: Kogan Page.

Hood, C. (1991) A public management for all seasons, *Public Administration*, **69**: 3–19.

Hunt, J. (1972) The foundation of a College. James Mackenzie lecture, *Journal of the Royal College of General Practitioners*, **23**: 5–20.

Hunter, D. (1992) Doctors as managers: poachers turned gamekeepers?, *Social Science and Medicine*, **35**: 557–66.

Hunter, D. (1993) *Rationing Dilemmas in Health Care*. London: NAHAT.

Hunter, D. (1995) Effective Practice, *Journal of Evaluation in Clinical Practice*, **1**: 131–4.

Hunter, D. (1998) Medicine, in M. Laffin (ed) *Beyond Bureaucracy? The Professions in the Contemporary Public Sector*. Aldershot: Ashgate.

Hurst, K., Harrison, S. and Ride, T. (2000) Primary care organisation and management: Evidence from a total purchasing pilot, *Journal of Management in Medicine*, **14**: 199–209.

Jeffreys, M. and Sachs, H. (1983) *Rethinking general practice*. London: Tavistock.

Johnson, T. (1972) *Professions and Power*. London: Macmillan.

Jost T. (1992) Recent developments in medical quality assurance and audit: An international comparative study, in R. Dingwall and P. Fenn (eds) *Quality and Regulation in Health Care: International Experiences*. London: Routledge.

Keen, J. and Packwood, T. (2000) Using case studies in health services and policy research, in *Qualitative Research in Health Care*, 2nd edn, C. Pope and N. Mays (eds.) London: BMJ Books.

Kerrison S., Packwood T. and Buxton M. (1993) Monitoring medical audit, in R. Robinson and J. Le Grand (eds.) *Evaluating the NHS Reforms*. London: King's Fund.

Klein, R. (1995) *The New Politics of the NHS*, 3rd edn. Harlow: Longman.

Klein, R. (1998) Can policy drive quality?, *Quality in Health Care*, 7: S51–S53.

Klein, R. (2001) Milburn's vision of a new NHS, *British Medical Journal*, 322: 1078–9.

Klein, R. and Maynard, A. (1998) On the way to Calvary, *British Medical Journal*, 317: 5.

Larkin, G. (1983) *Occupational Monopoly and Modern Medicine*. London: Tavistock Publications.

Le Grand, J. (1993) Evaluating the NHS Reforms, in R. Robinson and J. Le Grand (eds) *Evaluating the NHS Reforms*. London: Kings Fund.

Lewis, J. (1998) The medical profession and the state: GPs and the GP contract in the 1960s and the 1990s, *Social Policy and Administration*, 32: 132–50.

Lewis, J. M. and Considine, M. (1999) Medicine, economics and agenda-setting, *Social Science and Medicine*, 48: 393–405.

Lewis, R. (2004) Back to the future, *British Medical Journal*, 329: 932–3.

Light, D. (1998) Is NHS purchasing serious? An American perspective, *British Medical Journal*, 316: 217–20.

Light, D. (1999) Here we go again: repeating implementation errors, *British Medical Journal*, 319: 616–18.

Light, D. (2001) Managed competition, governmentality and institutional response in the United Kingdom, *Social Science and Medicine*, 52: 1167–81.

Lindblom, C. (1977) *Politics and Markets*. New York: Basic Books.

Lipman, T. (2000) The future general practitioner: out of date and running out of time, *British Journal of General Practice*, 50: 743–6.

Lukes, S. (1974) *Power: A Radical View*. Basingstoke: Macmillan.

Maheswaran, S. and Appleby, J. (1992) Building quality standards into contracts, *Health Direct*, September, 6–7.

Mahmood, K. (2001) Clinical governance and professional restratification in general practice, *Journal of Management in Medicine*, 15: 242–52.

Mark, A. (1991) Where are the medical managers?, *Journal of Management in Medicine*, 5: 6–12.

Mark, A. and Scott, H. (1992) Management in the National Health Service, in L. Wilcocks and J. Harrow (eds) *Rediscovering Public Services Management*. London: McGraw-Hill.

Marshall, M. N. (1999) How well do GPs and hospital consultants work together? A survey of the professional relationship, *Family Practice*, **16**: 33–8.

Maxwell, R. (1984) Quality assessment in health, *British Medical Journal*, **288**: 1470–72.

Mays, N., Goodwin N., Bevan G. and Wyke S. (1997) What is total purchasing?, *British Medical Journal*, **315**: 652–5.

McKee, M. and Clarke, A. (1995) Guidelines, enthusiasms, uncertainty, and the limits to purchasing, *British Medical Journal*, **310**: 101–4.

McKeown, T. (1979) *The Role of Medicine: Dream, Mirage or Nemesis?* Oxford: Blackwell.

Mechanic, D. (1991) Sources of countervailing power of medicine, *Journal of Health Politics, Policy and Law*, **16**: 485–506.

Merrison, A. (1979) *Report of the Royal Commission on the National Health Service*, Cmnd. 7615. London: HMSO.

Merrison Report (1975) *Report of the Committee of Inquiry into the Regulation of the Medical Profession*, Cmnd 6018. London: HMSO.

Millerson G. (1964) Dilemmas of professionalism, *New Society*, **88** (4 June): 15–16.

Ministry of Health (1962) *National Health Service: A Hospital Plan for England and Wales*, Cmnd. 1604. London: HMSO.

Ministry of Health (1966) *Report of the Committee on Senior Nursing Staff Structure*. London: HMSO.

Ministry of Health (1967) *First Report of the Joint Working Party on the Organisation of Medical Work in Hospitals*. London: HMSO.

Minogue, M. (2000) Should flawed models of public management be exported? Issues and practices. *Public Policy and Management Working Paper Series*, Working paper 15. Manchester: Institute for Development Policy and Management.

Moore, G. (1990) Doctors as managers: frustrating tensions, in D. Costain (ed) *The Future of Acute Services: Doctors as Managers*. London: King's Fund.

Moore, L. and Dalziel, M. (1993) Making the internal market work: a case for managed change, *British Medical Journal*, **307**: 1270–72.

Muhr, T. (1997) *Atlas.ti*. Berlin: Scientific Software Development.

National Audit Office (1987) *Competitive Tendering for Support Services in the National Health Service*, HC 318. London: HMSO.

National Health Service Executive (1994) *Quality and Contracting: Taking the Agenda Forward*. Leeds: NHSE.

National Health Service Executive (1995) *Acting on Complaints, the Government's Proposals to 'Being Heard'*. Leeds: NHSE.

National Health Service Executive (1998) *Annual Report*. Leeds: NHSE.

Navarro, V. (1976) Social class, political power, and the state and their implications in medicine, *Social Science and Medicine*, **10**: 437–56.

Navarro, V. (1977) *Medicine and Capitalism*. London: Croom Helm.

Navarro, V. (1978) *Class Struggle, the State and Medicine*. Oxford: Robertson.

Niskanen, W. (1971) *Bureaucracy and Representative Government*. Chicago: Aldine Atherton.

North, N. (1995) Alford revisited: The professional monopolisers, corporate rationalisers, community and markets, *Policy and Politics*, **23**: 115–25.

North, N. (1998) Implementing Strategy: The politics of healthcare commissioning, *Policy and Politics*, **26**: 5–14.

North, N., Lupton, C. and Khan, P. (1999) Going with the grain? General practitioners and the new NHS, *Health and Social Care*, **7**: 408–16.

North, N. and Peckham, S. (2001) Analysing structural interests in primary care groups, *Social Policy and Administration*, **35**: 426–40.

North of England Study of Standards and Performance in General Practice (1992) Medical Audit in General Practice, *British Medical Journal*, **304**: 1480–84.

Nuffield Provincial Hospitals Trust (1946) *The Hospital Surveys: The Doomsday Book of the Hospital Services*. Oxford: Oxford University Press.

Øvretveit, J. (1992) *Health Service Quality: An Introduction to Quality Methods for Health Services*. Oxford: Blackwell Scientific Publications.

O'Connor, J. (1973) *The Fiscal Crisis of the State*. New York: St Martin's Press.

Onion, C., Dutton, T., Walley, T., Turnbull, C., Dunne, W. and Buchan, I. Local clinical guidelines: description and evaluation of a participative method for their development and implementation, *Family Practice*, **13**: 28–34.

Packwood, T., Keen, J. and Buxton, M. (1991) *Hospitals in Transition: The Resource Management Experiment*. Milton Keynes: Open University Press.

Parry, N. and Parry, J. (1976) *The Rise of the Medical Profession*. London: Croom Helm.

Paton, C. (1990) The Prime Minister's Review of the NHS and the 1989 White Paper *Working for Patients*, in C. Ungerson and N. Manning (eds) *Social Policy Review*. Harlow: Longman.

Paton, C. (1998) *Competition and Planning in the NHS*. Cheltenham: Stanley Thornes.

Pettigrew, A., Ferlie, E. and McKee, L. (1992) *Shaping Strategic Change*. London: Sage.

Pilgrim D. and Rogers A. (1993) *A Sociology of Mental Health and Illness*. Buckingham: Open University Press.

Political and Economic Planning (1937) *Report on the British Health Services*. London: Political and Economic Planning.

Pollitt, C. (1993a) The struggle for quality: the case of the National Health Service, *Policy and Politics*, **21**: 161–70.

Pollitt, C. (1993b) The politics of medical quality: Auditing doctors in the UK and the USA, *Health Services Management Research*, **6**: 24–34.

Pollitt, C., Harrison, S., Hunter, D. J. and Marnoch, G. (1990) No hiding place: on the discomforts of researching the contemporary policy process, *Journal of Social Policy*, **19**: 169–190.

Power, M. (1997) *The Audit Society: Rituals of Verification*. Oxford: Oxford University Press.

Ranade, W. (1994) *A Future for the NHS? Health Care in the 1990s*. London: Longman.

Ranade, W. (1997). *A Future for the NHS? Health Care for the Millennium*. London: Longman.

Robinson, J. (1998) From contracts to service agreements: what can be learned from total purchasing?, *Journal of Management in Medicine*, **12**: 370–77.

Robinson, R. and Le Grand, J. (1993) *Evaluating the NHS Reforms*. London: King's Fund.

Robinson, R. and Stiener, A. (1998) *Managed Health Care*. Buckingham: Open University Press.

Royal College of General Practitioners (1985) *Quality in General Practice*. London: Royal College of General Practitioners.

Report of the Royal Commission on the NHS (1979) Cmnd 7615. London: HMSO.

Salter, B. (1994) Change in the British National Health Service: Policy paradox and the rationing issue, *International Journal of Health Services*, **24**(1): 45–72.

Salter, B. (1998) *The Politics of Change in the Health Service.* Basingstoke: Macmillan.

Smith, J. and Barnes, M. (2000) Developing primary care groups in the NHS: Towards diversity or uniformity?, *Public Money and Management*, January–March.

Smith, J., Regen, E., Shapiro, J. and Baines, D. (2000) National evaluation of general practitioner commissioning pilots: Lessons for Primary Care Groups, *British Journal of General Practice*, **50**: 469–72.

Smith, R. (1998) All changed, utterly changed, *British Medical Journal*, **316**: 1917–18.

Smith, R. (1999) Managing the clinical performance of doctors, *British Medical Journal*, **319**: 1314–15.

Somerset, M., Faulkner, A., Shaw, A., Dunn, L. and Sharp, D. (1999) Obstacles on the path to a primary-care led National Health Service: complexities of outpatient care, *Social Science and medicine*, **48**: 213–25.

South East Thames Regional Health Authority (1993) *Talking About Quality: Healthcare Quality Developments in South East Thames.* Bexhill-on-Sea: South Thames Regional Health Authority.

Spurgeon, P. (1993) Regulation or Free Market for the NHS, in I. Tilley (ed.) *Managing the Internal Market*. London: Paul Chapman Publishing.

Stevens, S. (2004) Reform strategies for the English NHS, *Health Affairs*, **23**: 37–44.

Strauss, A. L. and Corbin, J. (1998) *Basics of Qualitative Research*, 2nd edn. Thousand Oaks: Sage.

Strong, P. and Robinson, J. (1990) *The NHS: Under New Management*. Milton Keynes: Open University Press.

Surrender, R. and Fitzpatrick, R. (1999) Will doctors manage? Lessons from general practices fundholding, *Policy and Politics*, **27**: 491–502.

Turner, B. S. (1987) *Medical Power and Social Knowledge*. London: Sage.

Wainwright, D. (1996) *Primary Care Led Commissioning in East Kent*. Canterbury: Centre for Health Services Studies, University of Kent.

Walshe, K. (2003) Foundation hospitals: a new direction for NHS reform?, *Journal of the Royal Society of Medicine*, **96**: 106–10.

Walshe, K., Smith, J., Dixon, J. *et al.* (2004) Primary care trusts, *British Medical Journal*, **329**: 871–2.

Warwicker, T. (1998) Managerialism and the British GP: the GP as manager and as managed, *Journal of Management in Medicine*, **12**: 331–48.

Whynes, D. and Reed, G. (1994) Fundholders' referral patterns and perceptions of service quality in hospital provision of elective general surgery, *British Journal of General Practice*, **44**: 557–60.

Wilding, P. (1982) *Professional Power and Social Welfare*. London: Routledge and Kegan Paul.

Wilkin, D., Gillam, S., and Leese, B. (2000) *The National Tracker Survey of Primary Care Groups and Trusts: Progress and challenges 1999/2000*. Manchester: The University of Manchester.

Willets, D. and Goldsmith, M. (1988) *Managed Health Care: A New System for a Better Health Service*. London: Centre for Policy Studies.

Williams, S. J. (2001) Sociological imperialism and the profession of medicine revisited: where are we now?, *Sociology of Health and Illness*, **23**: 135–58.

Williamson, C. (1992) *Whose Standards? Consumer and Professional Standards in Health Care*. Buckingham: Open University Press.

Wyke, S., Malbon, G., McLeod, H., Posnett, J., Raftery, J. and Robinson, R. (1999) *Developing Primary Care in the New NHS: Lessons from Total Purchasing*. London: King's Fund.

Yin, R. (1994) *Case Study Research*. Thousand Oaks: Sage.

INDEX

Related books from Open University Press

Purchase from www.openup.co.uk or order through your local bookseller

CULTURES FOR PERFORMANCE IN HEALTH CARE

Russell Mannion, Huw T.O. Davies and Martin N. Marshall

- What is organizational culture?
- Do organizational cultures influence the performance of health-care organizations?
- Are organizational cultures capable of being managed to beneficial effect?

Recent legislation in the United Kingdom has led to significant reforms within the health-care system. Clinical quality, safety and performance have been the focus for improvement alongside systematic changes involving decision-making power being devolved to patients and frontline staff. However, as this book shows, improvements in performance are intrinsically linked to cultural changes within health-care settings.

Using theories from a wide range of disciplines, including economics, management and organization studies, policy studies and the health sciences, this book sets out definitions of cultures and performance, in particular the specific characteristics that help or hinder performance. Case studies of high- and low-performing hospital trusts and primary care trusts are used to explore the links between culture and performance. These studies provide examples of strategies to create beneficial, high-performance cultures that may be used by other managers. Moreover, implications for future policies and research are outlined.

Cultures for Performance in Health Care is essential reading for those with an interest in health-care management and health policy, including students, researchers, policy makers and health-care professionals.

Contents

Series editor's introduction – List of figures and tables – List of boxes – About the authors – Foreword 1 by Aidan Halligan and Jay Bevington – Foreword 2 by Nigel Edwards – Acknowledgements – Introduction: policy background and overview – Making sense of organizational culture in health care – Does organizational culture influence health-care performance? A review of existing evidence – Culture and performance in acute hospital trusts: integration and synthesis of case-study evidence – Culture and performance in English acute hospital trusts: condensed case study narratives – Findings from a quantitative analysis of all English NHS acute trusts – Findings from the primary care case studies – Summary, conclusions and implications for policy and research – Appendix 1 Research design and methods of data gathering and analysis – Appendix 2 Quantitative models and data definitions – References – Appendices.

256pp   0 335 21553 X (Paperback)   0 335 21554 8 (Hardback)

COMPARATIVE HEALTH POLICY IN THE ASIA-PACIFIC

Robin Gauld (ed)

Based upon research from eight countries in the Asia-Pacific – Australia, China, Hong Kong, Japan, New Zealand, Singapore, South Korea, Taiwan – this book analyses and compares their differing health policies. Key issues the book probes include:

- The ways that health care is financed and delivered across the region
- The historical and institutional arrangements that impact upon health policy and health care
- How the health systems differ between the countries under study
- How policymakers and service providers deal with unlimited demand and limited funding and issues such as service coverage and quality
- How pharmaceuticals and population health strategies are managed
- What the roles of the state and various other players (such as the private sector and professional associations) are in the making of health policy and delivery of health care
- The challenges that lie ahead for health care and health policy in the region

Comparative Health Policy in the Asia-Pacific is key reading for students, researchers and policy makers with an interest in health policy. It is relevant to those studying medicine and health studies, anthropology, history, sociology, public policy, politics and Asian studies.

Contributors
Michael Barr, Gerald Bloom, Tung-Liang Chiang, Stephen Duckett, Robin Gauld, Derek Gould, Naoki Ikegami, Soonman Kwon.

Contents
List of contributors – Acknowledgements – Abbreviations – Introduction – China – South Korea – Taiwan – Australia – Japan – Singapore – Hong Kong – New Zealand – Conclusion – Index.

256pp   0 335 21433 9 (Paperback)   0 335 21434 7 (Hardback)

HEALTH CARE COVERAGE DETERMINATIONS

Timothy Jost (ed)

"A ground breaking set of case studies about how [health care] coverage decisions are made".

> Robert A. Berenson, M.D., Senior Fellow at the Urban Institute, Washington D.C. and former Director of the Center for Health Plans and Providers of the US Medicare program.

Developed countries are facing rapidly rising health care costs and one of the major factors driving health care cost growth is the continual development and diffusion of new, generally more expensive, health care technologies.

This book contains:

- A description of the institutions, procedures and criteria used by eight countries for assessing technologies for public insurance coverage.
- An analysis of the role of interest groups, and of the public interest, in these decision making processes
- An examination of how particular technologies are treated differently by different countries, and why.

Based upon research from Australia, Canada, Germany, The Netherlands, Spain, Switzerland, the United States of America and the United Kingdom, the contributors argue that although each of these countries is committed to evidence-based scientific assessment of technologies, in fact adoption of technologies is significantly affected by political considerations, and in particular by the influence of interest groups. Moreover, it offers recommendations as to how technology assessment for coverage policy can be improved to serve better the public interest.

Health Care Coverage Determinations is essential reading for health policy makers, managers, researchers and students with an interest in health economics, health care provision and the politics affecting health care legislation.

Contributors

Liliana Bulfone, Tanisha Carino, Peter C. Coyte, Anna García-Altés, Colleen M. Flood, Stefan Greb, Felix Gurtner, Anthony Harris, Timothy Stoltzfus Jost, Eric Nauenberg, Christopher Newdick, Dea Niebuhr, Guillaume Roduit, Heinz Rothgang, Frans F.H. Rutten, Dominique Sprumont, Juergen Wasem.

Contents

List of Contributors – Introduction – Getting Value for Money: The Australian Experience – A Complex Taxonomy: Technology Assessment in Canadian Medicare – Evaluating New Health Technology in the English National Health Service – Benefit Decisions in German Social Insurance – Health Care Coverage in the Netherlands: The Dutch Drug Reimbursement System (GVS) – Health Care Coverage Determinations in Spain – Health Care Coverage Determinations in Switzerland – The Medicare Coverage Determination Process in the United States – What Can We Learn From Our Country Studies? – Conclusion – Index.

224pp   0 335 21495 9 (Paperback)   0 335 21496 7 (Hardback)

HEALTH POLICY AND ECONOMICS
CHALLENGES AND OPPORTUNITIES
Peter C. Smith, Laura Ginnelly and Mark Sculpher

Health economics has made major contributions to the development of health policy in many countries. This book describes those successes and looks forward to the major contributions that health economics can bring to bear on emerging policy issues in health and health care.

With contributions from internationally recognized researchers, this book addresses generic policy issues confronting health systems across the developed world. The coverage progresses from micro, patient level issues to macro, whole system issues including:

- Determining cost-effective treatments
- Fair distribution of health care
- Regulatory issues such as performance measurement and incentives
- Revenue distribution
- Decentralization and internationalization of health systems

Health Policy and Economics identifies the major contributions that health economics makes to important policy issues in health and health care. It is key reading for policy makers and health managers as well as students and academics with an interest in health policy and health services research.

Contributors
Ron L. Akehurst, Karen E. Bloor, Martin Buxton, Karl P. Claxton, Richard Cookson, Diane A. Dawson, Paul Dolan, Mike Drummond, Brian Ferguson, Hugh Gravelle, Maria Goddard, Katharina Hauck, John Hutton, Andrew M. Jones, Rowena Jacobs, Paul Kind, Rosella Levaggi, Guillem López Casanovas, Alan K. Maynard, Nigel Rice, Anthony Scott, Rebecca Shaw, Trevor Sheldon, Andrew D. Street, Mark Sculpher, Matthew Sutton, Peter C. Smith, Adrian Towse, Aki Tsuchiya, Alan H. Williams.

Contents
List of contributors – Series editor's introduction – Acknowledgements – Introduction – Its just evaluation for decision-making: Recent developments in, and challenges for, cost-effectiveness research – Valuing health outcomes: Ten questions for the insomniac health economist – Eliciting equity-efficiency trade-offs in health – Using longitudinal data to investigate socioeconomic inequality in health – Regulating health care markets – Efficiency measurement in health care: Recent developments, current practice and future research – Incentives and the UK medical labour market – Formula funding of health purchasers: towards a fairer distribution? – Decentralization in health care: Lessons from public economics – European integration and the economics of health care – Health economics and health policy: A postscript – Index.

312pp   0 335 21574 2 (Paperback)   0 335 21575 0 (Hardback)

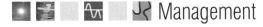
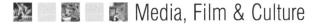
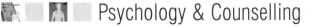
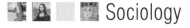
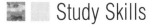
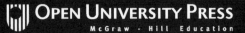
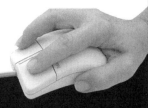